Occipital

Explained

Migraines

Occipital Headaches, Neuralgia
Symptoms, Occipital Nerve, Neuralgia
in Head, Facial Neuralgia, Occipital
Neuralgia Symptoms, Neuralgia
Treatment, Neuralgic Pain, Occipital
Neuralgia Treatment, All Covered

Published by Cleal Publishing

Copyright ©2017 Cleal Publishing

ISBN (978-0-9955610-3-8)

Disclaimer

While the author and publisher have made all available efforts to ensure the information contained in this book was correct as of press time, neither the author nor publisher assumes and hereby disclaims any liability to any party for damages, disruption, or loss caused by the use and application, directly or indirectly, of any information presented including any errors. This book is not meant to substitute for medical advice from a qualified healthcare professional. The reader should regularly consult with a healthcare professional in matters relating to his/her health, particularly with respect to any of the symptoms discussed that may require professional treatment. The accuracy and completeness of information provided herein and opinions stated herein are not guaranteed or warranted to produce any particular results, and the advice and strategies contained herein may not be suitable for every individual.

Contents

Chapter1 Headaches 5

  Headache (Cephalalgia) 5

  Types of headaches 10

Chapter 2 Neuralgia 24

  Head neuralgies 29

Chapter 3 Occipital nerves anatomy 35

Chapter 4 Occipital headaches and pain in the back of the head 43

  Occipital neuralgia. How many people have this type of headache? 48

  Etiology. How and why does the occipital neuralgia develop? 49

Chapter 5 Occipital neuralgia symptoms 53

Chapter 6 Diagnosing occipital neuralgia 58

Chapter 7 Occipital neuralgia and the differential diagnosis 64

Chapter 8 Occipital neuralgia treatment 70

  Medical (pharmacological) treatment 70

  General nerve blocks 76

  Surgical procedures 81

    Decompression tecnhniques and liberation of nerves 82

    Rhizotomy and neurectomy surgery 85

    Ganglioneurectomy 86

    Radiofrequency ganglio-neurectomy (RFGN),pulsed radiofrequency ablation (PRA) treatment 87

    Occipital nerve stimulator(ONS) 90

  Non surgical treatments 93

    Cryotherapy and cryoablation 93

Botulinum toxin A injection (Botox A, BoNT-A)............................ 94

Phenol (alcohol) block 96

Physical therapy.. 97

Warm compresses 100

B vitamin nutrition supplement 100

Acupuncture or dry needling...................................... 101

Cognitive behavioral therapy and psychological consultations
involving pain and treatment 102

Chapter 9 Prevention 103

Works Cited 107

Do not undervalue the headache. While it is at its sharpest it seems a bad investment; but when relief begins, the unexpired remainder is worth $4 a minute.

Mark Twain (1835-1910)

INTRODUCTION

Occipital neuralgia originates from damage to the occipital nerves that arise from the spinal cord upward and innervate the skin and muscles of the top and back of the head. Even though pain in the back of the head may indicate other problems, it usually develops for unknown reasons. The symptoms are, however, disabling in everyday life and may interfere with the ability to function at work, and can affect relations with family, as well as mood and sleep. It is important to mention that these headaches have a good prognosis and treatments have proved to work and eliminate in even the severest cases.

Even when you feel that your pain doesn't leave you, learn to appreciate the days without the pain. Understandably, hours and days with a headache may make you choose the activities that you are able to perform and those you aren't capable of at the moment, which could lead you to disappoint yourself and others. The good days will come and pain will change with something else in your life. The treatment advice and prevention are here to help you battle with such troubling times. However, this isn't a substitute for a serious and warm conversation with your doctor when you have any perplexity about your health and pain.

Chapter 1. Headaches

Headache (Cephalalgia)

Headaches are the most common symptom that is severe enough to interfere with normal daily functions. Headaches may appear for various reasons. They may be provoked for even more reasons. A headache is a common reaction to a generalized problem that confronts our bodies. They are an alarm set off by a terrible state of hydration, lack of electrolytes, nutrients level, or perhaps an infection. Since it is a very common symptom, not every man or woman shares his/her story of a headache with a general practitioner. And a headache may mean so many things.

Some headaches are mild, usually described as tension or discomfort, and they rarely affect on person's abilities, while others vary from moderate to severe and very severe, which means an emergency condition. Some people have struggles with headaches daily, and some of them several times a month. Most headaches are easily treated with analgesics (pain killers), which is usually the beginning of the treatment. However, these medications do not cure the headache, but only hide it. It is important to try to find out what is behind it. 90% of people reported that they had a headache at least once in their lifetime, and 50% of world population has headaches throughout the year depending on the type of headache. (1)

Headaches are either primary or secondary, depending on the cause. Migraine, tension, and cluster headaches belong to the primary headache disorders because of their unclear pathophysiology, benign nature, and tendency to chronicity. Many headaches fall into this category of unknown causes. Secondary headaches develop for clear reasons, and may even progress to a fatal outcome. Pain may come from various organs, structures and nerves in the face, skull, and neck. This is usually characteristic of secondary headaches. A headache can appear suddenly or develop gradually over the years. Sudden headaches are sometimes cause for alarm. They can be a sign of a sudden rupture of blood vessel in the head and bleeding, or a complication after a serious injury to the head or infection. When this happens, a person usually experiences some other symptoms as well: nausea, vomiting, light and sound nuisance, convulsions, loss of consciousness, or amnesia. These are emergency conditions that require immediate attention. If a person doesn't receive immediate help, he/she will continue to collect blood in the skull, which isn't able to provide more space for such an amount of blood and tissue. Accordingly, the brain begins to compress the sensitive structures in the neck, which are vital centers for regulation of breathing and heart functions. This may end fatally. Other headaches can be classified as subacute and chronic. They are long-lasting and have a better prognosis. However, they play an important role in professional and personal life and functioning.

The third group of headaches, which is distinct from the previous two, is a headache caused by neuropathic pain. Many nerve plexuses spread from the brain to important structures. The head and neck are a part of the body where there are many muscles, tendons, blood vessels, bones, and glands, all contained in a complex but strong and organized construction. If any of these parts affects the function of the other, in such a tight space, problems may occur. This happens when the nerves become pressed and injured.

There are several types of headaches with different symptoms and location of the pain, associated symptoms, severity, and provoking factors. We can also classify the type of headache a person has based on some factors such as gender, age, profession, lifestyle, provoking factors, and genetic predisposition.

By intensity

Mild – the pain is only noticeable and is easily relieved with NSAIDs.

Moderate – the pain affects on person in daily functioning, is sharp or dull, and it is either long-lasting or it returns in the form of episodes.

Severe – pain is making it difficult for a person to drive and stay concentrated; sometimes there are other symptoms.

Very severe – pain is unbearable, person is in great distress, loses huge amounts of energy, and is weak.

By gender and age

Some types of headaches are more frequent in women and some in men. In history, headaches were more often linked to women and their different social roles, stress, and probably hysteria. However, these allusions proved to be untrue and headaches are at the moment equally present in men and women, which sometimes can be connected to hormonal disbalance and sometimes not. According to many scientific studies, migraine is linked to estrogen hormone, so it appears more frequently in women, especially in the generative period with hormone fluctuations. As the estrogen becomes lower when menstrual bleeding begins, the headache begins too. This is referred to as the menstrual migraine. However, when estrogen is low, there are possibilities for the development of a migrainous headache. Migraine bouts also last longer and have higher intensity than in men. Also, associated migrainous symptoms, such as light sensitivity and nausea, are more frequently reported by women. Cluster headache is more frequent in young people, or at least those under the age of 40 years. It is two to three times more common in men, too. These types of headaches are the strong ones, the ones that can make a man hit his head against the wall. There is no known reason why there would be higher prevalence in men. Other types of headaches have no difference in age and gender. When it comes to neuralgia, reports are often incomplete. The prevalence of neuralgia in women is somewhat higher, even though many studies concluded that there is an equal prevalence.

By eating habits, lifestyle and genetic and family influences

It has been proven by various studies that some foods may induce headaches. These are the foods that most people find delicious or difficult to avoid: cheese, fish, chocolate and wine. In these foods and drinks, there is a substance called tyramine that is known to induce headaches. When tyramine enters the blood stream, it affects the blood vessels, which provokes migrainous pain. It is helpful if people who have frequent headaches avoid these drinks and foods. But some people report to their doctors that the headache didn't start until a couple of hours or even a day after they ate these foods. Nevertheless, it may be useful to keep a diary about foods that caused headaches and the provoking ones that actually didn't cause it. This phenomenon is usually seen in people with migraine, primarily headaches, that are linked to pathophysiology with the state of blood vessels before and during the migrainous bout. The reaction to a certain food is individual, and one person may react severely to one type of food while someone else doesn't. It is probably best not to test those theories by self-inducing headaches. Some food additives may also induce such a reaction, and not just the tyramine.

Another factor that contributes to the development of migraine and other headaches is nicotine. A cluster headache episode may be provoked in people who have been smokers for many years. Discontinuing the use of nicotine, however, brings no improvement. Nicotine induces constriction to the blood vessels, most importantly in the brain, and it also stimulates the nerves of the head, and increases the sensitivity to pain contributing to the headache. Studies show that non-smokers have headaches less frequently, and that smokers have headaches that seem to last 14 days each month, varying in intensity. Cluster headaches have been firmly linked to smoking and they don't seem to vanish after cessation of smoking. The smoking effect is also evident in people who are passive smokers. Other theories are that smokers tend to have less oxygen bound to their red blood cells, and have a higher level of carbon monoxide, which can be manifested by headaches, and also they have increased metabolism in degradation of pain medication. (2)

Alcohol use has also been found to be a contributing factor to headaches, and not only huge amounts of alcohol. Wine and beer have been scientifically proven to have tyramine in small amounts that can trigger a migrainous headache. Alcohol may, however, trigger tension-type headaches, cluster headaches, and some other less common types of headaches. It is widely known that headaches appear as an accompanying sign of the hangover, among other symptoms. It appears because of the dehydration and low blood sugar, but as a consequence of alcohol's toxic effects too. Chronic alcohol use may develop not only the illness of the liver but also B vitamin deficiency. B vitamin is very important in regeneration of nerves.

Professional stress, especially chronic stress, may affect the development of headaches. Stress influences blood vessels and muscles of the head, making them constricted and stiff, which then causes the headache we call a tension type of headache. People under great psychological stress tend to have enhanced sensitivity to pain and sensitization of nerves of the muscles or central nervous system. This is called somatization and it often remains unexplained. Stress induces tension of the muscles and tendons of the scalp. This comes from an abnormal position we take each time we are under stress. The position is defensive and muscles become stiffer and contracted. Thus the blood vessels responsible for the blood supply become compressed and induce more stiffness and pain. This also includes neck muscles that become inflamed after a long time in an uncomfortable position. Neuralgia and neuropathy may increase in intensity with anxious thoughts and stress, which is especially important to either eliminate the severest pain or to perform any method of relaxation.

Family factor and genetics may also be responsible; these factors may have only a little influence or none at all. Cluster and migraine headaches are usually present in other members of family as well.

Types of headaches
1. Migraine
2. Tension headache
3. Cluster headache
4. Headache due to injury
5. Headache due to vascular disorder
6. Non-vascular headache, increased pressure in the head
7. Toxications or withdrawal syndromes
8. Infections
9. Headache due to hypertension or other illnesses
10. Pain that originates from nose, eyes, ears, throat, teeth
11. Unspecified headaches
12. Somatization headache
13. Neuropathies and neuralgias (including trigeminal neuropathy and occipital neuralgia)

Primary headaches:

1. Migraine

Migraine is the most common type of headache, most commonly affecting the female population. Estrogen has been shown to be a factor in the development of migraine, especially when it fluctuates in the generative period, that is, until the menopause. When estrogen becomes low during a woman's menstrual cycle, headaches may occur. The fluctuation and sudden decrease have been shown to be responsible, but with unknown mechanism. Even though men also have estrogen, their level stays low through the whole lifetime. Besides the estrogen, other factors include lifestyle, some habits, ingestion of some foods, beer, or red wine. In its core pathophysiology, there is a change in the blood vessels of the brain due to hyperstimulation of the brain cortex, which then spreads to all structures of the brain and its blood vessels, thus increasing the sensitivity to pain and spreading in the area of the trigeminal nerve. The tendency to have migraine and hyperstimulated cortex of brain is genetic. Some don't agree with this theory, and there are other theories, but they all agree on treating the consequences of such uncertain mechanism: a one-sided headache which is only responsive to one type of treatment. (3)

"Migraine" comes from the Greek word *hemicranios*, which means half of the head, since migraine pain is, in most cases, located on one half of the head. The pain is dull, pulsating, and spreading. A migrainous episode goes through four stages: prodrome, aura, headache, postdrome.

A migraine may present with or without an "aura." The aura is a complex of symptoms that appears a couple of days or hours before the real headache begins. It is always a sign that a headache is about to develop with pain that increases more and more. Symptoms of an aura are nausea, vomiting, light and sound sensitivity, confusion, fatigue, flashes and dots in the eyesight, tingling in one part of the body. These may also be accompanying signs along with the headache. The headache is usually one-sided, localized in the temporal region, above the earlobe with pain that can spread to the eye and is pulsing or throbbing. It is speculated that a migraine actually originates from damage to the trigeminal nerve, which is responsible for innervation of sensitivity of the face. Even though symptoms do appear as a trigeminal neuropathic disorder, some other factors are included as well: low serotonin level, hormonal disbalance, eating habits, environmental changes, etc. Pain may last untreated for 72 hours and then it slowly decreases in intensity. People who know about their migraine will act fast as soon as the first symptoms appear, no matter how light they are and how mild the pain is. Some of the accompanying symptoms may last even in the convalescent period. It is treated with specific antimigrainous therapy. Therapy is focused on preventing the episodes of pain and treatment as well. Therapy consists of pain-killers, triptans, ergotamine, and other symptom-specific drugs.

2. Tension-type headache (TTP)

TTP is a very common type of headache and is reported more often by women than men. This condition is a pain that affects people who are under great stress. They complain about such typical symptoms as pressure and pain in the head in a shape of a band around their head that presses on the head. Other than stress, it may develop because of the bad posture during working hours and anxiety. Situations that provoke it are extreme light, noise, and dehydration. Tension-type headaches are classified as a primary group of headaches, without any serious cause, and with good prognosis, but a tendency to chronicity. They are considered to be linked with anxiety, stress, increased pain perception, and probably a somatoform disorder. It may be associated with other similar channeled symptoms, as well.

The pain lasts a minimum of 30 minutes and a maximum of a couple of hours. It may be mild or severe. Pain is usually dull and pressuring. The surface of the head, i.e., the muscles of the head are stiff. Tension headache is caused by abnormal contraction of scalp muscles, which then compromises the blood circulation and induces pain. The skin of the head is very tender to touch. The tension headache may be episodic, when it appears once per month, or chronic, when it is present for more than three months, with more than days when the headache is present. It is treated with acetaminophen and non-steroid anti-inflammatory drugs and with relaxation methods as well as cognitive behavioral therapy. Some recommend acupuncture.

3. Cluster headache

Cluster headaches are probably the severest headaches a person can experience. The pain is so strong that a person would do anything to stop the pain, even hit his head on the wall. It is more prevalent in men than women. There are episodic and chronic cluster headaches. Episodic cluster headache is characteristic for intermittent headaches and painless periods, which may last even 30 days. The pain appears in the same season of the year, every year. Chronic cluster headache is rarer than episodic and appears in 10% of the people who have cluster headaches. The period without headache is shorter than 30 days, which makes it more difficult to handle with.

Cluster headaches appear in many episodes intermittently with periods without pain, but also with great fear about the next episode. The headaches are very intensive and usually one-sided. Pain begins at the area around one eye and then spreads over the whole side of the face. The pain might become sharp and pulsating and within 5 to 10 minutes it becomes very severe and unbearable. It lasts for a maximum of 90 minutes and then leaves. However, the next episode will start on the same day, and a person doesn't know when that next attack might happen. This type of headache is very rare. Before another attack happens, a person may notice some symptoms that foretell the headache; among them are swollen eyes, dilated pupils, paleness, sweating on the face, nervousness, red eye, tearing, runny nose, drooping eyelid, etc., and they might give time to prepare somewhat for it. These symptoms continue as the pain progresses. Cluster headaches appear for unknown reasons and are rare, but there are theories about development from hypothalamus disorder or its being triggered by alcohol or nitroglycerin. The hypothalamus is an important structure in the middle of the brain that secretes hormones that regulate the function of other glands and substances responsible for the constriction of blood vessels. This may be somehow connected to cluster headache and its intensity.

It is sometimes difficult to differentiate a cluster headache from a migraine, since they both affect one side of the head. People with cluster headache also have trouble with sinuses, but these are not due to respiratory infections but rather because of the stimulation of the nerves that lie around them. Treatment consists of special measures, because ordinary pain treatment has no effect. Even

though it involves severe pain, the cluster headache is benign and
without any structural cause. (4)

Secondary headaches:

4. Headache that follows an injury

A headache can develop as a complication of an injury,
even from the slightest blow to the head. As the first signs of
damage to the brain, confusion and amnesia appear. If a person
can reconstruct the event prior or at the time of the trauma, it is
likely that there is a functional damage to the brain, at least. These
conditions develop suddenly and within 24 hours after the trauma.
The person needs to be immediately examined by a doctor, so the
best idea is to visit the nearest emergency center for necessary
assessment and observation. When the structures inside the head
are injured, they begin to swell and, since the skull is enclosed
with bones, this swelling begins to pressure other tissue as well,
possibly causing damage. Symptoms may vary, depending on the
nature of the injury and trauma. Headache may become similar to
a tension-type headache, as a band around the head, or affect only
one side. Some headaches are just functional and will soon
diminish, but some can be serious. Associated symptoms, besides
confusion and amnesia, include watery nose (which is actually
liquid from inside the brain) or leakage from ears, buzzing in the
ears, changes in blood pressure, light and sound sensitivity,
nausea, vomiting, shallow breathing, seizures, and loss of
consciousness. When the injury is mild, the person is advised to
be observed and should possibly take some medication; if the
injury to the head was very severe, there is a need for immediate
surgery. Sometimes headaches may last for years after the trauma,
and studies show that there are some psychological factors
included that influence the amplified perception of pain. The
treatment is with NSAIDs, antidepressants, anticonvulsives, and
psychological and relaxational approaches, which, all taken
together, may not help enough after all.

5. Headaches due to vascular disorder

Headaches may precede some important vascular events. These are actually headaches that appear in a condition called transitory ischemic attack (TIA), which is also referred to as a mini-stroke. TIA is a warning event of the possible stroke and should be taken seriously. It is a condition that develops from lack of circulation through one part of the brain. TIA lasts from 30 to 60 minutes and may manifest with vision problems, possible one-eyed blindness, trouble speaking, numbness or tingling in one part of the body, problems with walking, loss of consciousness, abnormal taste and smell, abnormality in the facial expression, problems with lifting arms and any other function with arms. TIA doesn't leave any damage to the brain, but is a cause for alarm, and indicates that the blood flow to the brain is limited. The next episode of cut circulation through the brain may be a stroke. The stroke may have the same symptoms, which aren't at first evident, so the best idea is to visit the nearest emergency center if some of these symptoms are noticed.

Inflammation in the arteries of the head may also induce headaches. The reason behind it may be an autoimmune reaction that attacks arteries of the surface of the head, often in the temporal region above the earlobe. This is characteristic for the older population. The most common arteritis is temporal arteritis, which affects the artery that spreads its branches on the side of the head. When it is inflamed, some symptoms become evident. Pain appears to be pulsating and one-sided, provoked by chewing and speaking. Treatment consists of specific therapy for autoimmune illnesses to modify the immunological response, usually with corticosteroids.

6. Non-vascular headache, i.e., increased intracranial pressure (ICP)

This headache appears because of the compression on the skull's inner structures The causes of increased ICP, besides injuries, could be tumors, infections, birth malformations, aneurysms, epilepsy, complications of high blood pressure, and others. However, the pain isn't always present, which is why these conditions, which could be fatal, often stay undetected. People don't experience any symptoms and therefore don't think that something is wrong until the symptoms gradually or suddenly appear. Then, a person experiences pain in the head, anywhere from the occiput to the forehead, depending on the location of the process, along with nausea and vomiting, vision problems, confusion, shallow breathing, seizures, loss of consciousness, and some other symptoms that occur because of the compression on the delicate structures of brain and brainstem in the neck-head junction. Treatment is usually surgical and urgent and has the goal of eliminating the cause of increased intracranial pressure.

7. Toxications, medications, and withdrawal syndromes

Toxins, medications, foreign plants, and fungi may also cause headaches. Among substances that may cause headaches are nitrogen oxide (NO), alcohol, cocaine, carbon monoxide, pollution gases, chemicals with strong smells, and toxins that have a direct toxic effect on the whole organism (pesticides, lead, copper, etc). They can be either inhaled or ingested or applied on the skin forming a generalized reaction with headache.

Some medications can cause headaches as a result of overuse. This happens with ergotamine, triptan, and almost every analgesic. After a substance has been used for a long time and the use suddenly stops, the body has been "used to" having that substance and doesn't tolerate it well when the substance isn't present. That is how the symptoms of withdrawal develop; they can include headache (substances include caffeine, opioid analgesics, estrogen therapy, and others). Pain medications are known to sometimes cause the withdrawal symptoms.

Headache may also be caused by some medications, including even painkillers such as NSAIDs, ergotamine, and triptans. This happens more often in women. The mechanism is that these medications are used too often and the body becomes tolerant to the standard dose, even though these medications do not induce addiction. Overuse is defined as use of analgesics for more than 15 days over a three-month period.

8. Infections

Infective agents such as bacteria or viruses may induce generalized symptoms, including headaches, which we are all very familiar with. Infections of the upper respiratory tract commonly manifest with respiratory symptoms, high fever, and headaches. Infections from the throat may spread to the brain layers (meninges), causing meningitis, which appears with high fever, sensitivity to light, nausea, vomiting, and a headache. Usually, these infections are bacterial, but they can also be viral, fungal, or parasitic. Infections of any part of the head (eye, ear, sinus, teeth, and even bones) may induce a headache. Infection of the maxillary sinus appears when the secretion from the nose spreads through the cavity to the upper jaw. This creates pain in the cheeks, eyes, and teeth, which can be associated with pain in the head. Deep sinuses also create specific deep pain in the center of the head. Some generalized infections may last for months and induce mild to severe headaches.

9. Headache due to hypertension or other illnesses

Some illnesses may induce a headache through a specific mechanism, depending on the nature of the illness. The most common chronic illness that causes headaches is hypertension, when, with a sudden rise in blood pressure, pain appears in the back of the head along with other symptoms, such as nose bleeding, nausea, redness of the face and neck, dizziness, or red spots in the eye. These signs may not be present with every increase in blood pressure, and often this is asymptomatic. This is important to mention, since many people rely on high pressure to appear always with a headache as a warning sign, which isn't obligatory and may be the reason why some people suddenly have a stroke.

Hypothyroidism (lowered function of the thyroid gland) may also be the cause of headaches. Cardiac or kidney disease, as well as conditions without proper air concentration of oxygen and high carbon dioxide, low blood sugar because of going a long time without taking any food, or high calcium in blood, which are not illnesses but rather special disorders caused by environmental changes, mostly can manifest first with a headache.

Tumors induce headache through various mechanisms, such as an increase of intracranial pressure or direct compression on some structures and the nerves. Depending on the location of the tumor, pain may appear in the back of the head, or in the forehead.

10. Pain that originates from nose, eyes, ears, throat, teeth, and other parts

The head is a part of our body where various important structures are placed and connected closely to each other. All of those structures may become ill, inflamed, or injured and thus may induce headache. This may be due to infections, injuries, or specific illnesses of each part; for example, glaucoma (increased pressure in the eye), vision problems and strabismus, foreign body in the ear or nose, decayed teeth, pain from the jaw joint, tumors that affect nerves, etc.

If a person develops damage or degeneration of the jaw joint, he/she may develop some severe headaches that are provoked by chewing and speaking. This type of headache is referred to as Costen syndrome. The most severe pain is in front and on the back side of the earlobe and spreading. Treatment can be surgical.

11. Unspecified headaches

Unspecified headaches may be included either in primary or secondary headaches, with known cause. Hypnic headache is a rare type of headache that appears for unknown reasons during the night, in sleep. This happens even more than 15 times during the night and lasts up to 15 minutes. It is characteristic of older people. The headache is one- or both-sided and appears more often in women. It is treated with specific medications, including lithium, which requires special attention, and some medications and substances that affect the blood vessels, such as topiramate and caffeine).

SUNCT syndrome is another nonspecified headache; this is an acronym for short-lasting unilateral neuralgiform attacks with conjunctival injection and tearing, which is actually a headache with eye symptoms. It may look similar to a cluster headache and trigeminal neuralgia, but it has a different duration and etiology. SUNCT is more a neuralgic syndrome but different from trigeminal neuralgia. However, the treatment includes antidepressants and anticonvulsives and shows little or no effect from neurological blocks. (5)

Eagle's syndrome is a condition in which a part of temporal bone, the styloid pointy process, is abnormally long and compresses the nerves of the area between the throat and ear, inducing pain in this region.

Orgasmic and preorgasmic headache is a headache that appears during sexual activity and is classified as a primary type of headache. The pain appears in the head and neck, which distinguishes it from the migraine. It is usually benign and pain relief comes with ordinary pain-killers, such as NSAIDs.

Hemiplegic headache is a rare condition where the central nervous system is not functioning properly and a person develops headaches and a temporary paralysis on one side of the body. Other symptoms may be the symptoms of aura: loss of balance, nausea, vomiting, light and sound sensitivity, double vision, problems with speech, etc. Scientific research has classified this as a type of migraine and a condition that is genetically influenced.

Ice pick headache is often described as being sharp, as if a needle or an ice pick has been inserted in the skull. The pain is sudden and on one side of the head. It may appear at night and wake the person. It is short lasting: After 5-30 seconds, the pain passes. This too belongs to the group of primary headaches, since there is no known cause that could explain their development. They are more likely to appear in people who already have some other type of headache, often a migraine.

Exercise headache appears during or after excessive exercise. It is also a primary headache. The pain is pulsating, throbbing, on one or both sides, and includes sound and light sensitivity, nausea, and vomiting. This headache may last from five minutes to 48 hours. The probable cause is sudden increase in blood pressure and pulse or dilation of blood vessels, which changes the blood flow to the brain. The exact cause is still unknown; these are only theories. It is more likely to appear after exercising under inappropriate conditions that induce dilation of blood vessels, such as high temperature of the environment or poor ventilation. Treatment with NSAIDs and the beta blocker propranolol shows good results. (4)

12. Somatization headache

This disorder, somatization, or somatoform disorder, appears as channeled psychological stress through physical ailments, meaning that a person complains about some pain or other symptoms if, after many diagnostic procedures, they aren't being explained. Thus these unexplained headaches are explained with psychological pathophysiology without any psychiatric disorder, which is a non-specific diagnosis with a specific treatment. The condition is complex, and usually the headache is associated with other symptoms, such as pain in other sites, gastrointestinal dysfunction, or difficulty with breathing. The whole clinical presentation doesn't correspond with any known medical condition and doesn't reveal the structural cause of the headache or any other symptoms, in fact. The headache may be different and some scientific research placed tension-type headaches into this group of symptoms. A person is usually constantly worried about the symptoms and because of the unknown diagnosis. Treatment is usually with medicines, cognitive behavioral therapy, and relaxation therapy. Cognitive behavioral therapy plays the key role. A person learns new behavior to handle stress, frustrations, and emotional expression principles. (6)

Third group of headaches: facial and occipital neuralgia

13. Neuropathies and neuralgias (including trigeminal neuropathy and occipital neuralgia)

Neuralgia is only a syndrome of pain due to nerve damage. Neuropathy is any damage to the nerve, which, as consequence has many different symptoms, usually problems with sensation. Both of them appear as a consequence of illness or damage to the nerve in any part of the body. Both of them may develop from the nerves of the head. These types of headaches appear because of damage to the nerves of the head and/or face. Therefore, we can say that there is a division between occipital and facial neuralgia. Both of them are present in the population, but facial neuralgia, especially trigeminal neuralgia is the most common. All of them include in their names the name of the nerve that is affected. Trigeminal neuralgia develops when the trigeminal nerve is damaged. There are several types of neuralgias:

- Trigeminal neuralgia
  o Primary trigeminal neuralgia
  o Symptomatic trigeminal neuralgia
- Glossopharyngeal
- Occipital neuralgia
- Supraorbital neuralgia
- Infraorbital neuralgia

There are some theories about why and how neuralgias develop, since the real mechanism isn't clear. There are theories of a purely peripheral cause, a purely central cause (due to an illness of the central nervous system), a peripheral origin with central mechanism (combined mechanism), or a combination of multiple factors. Usually the actual reason isn't found with any diagnostic procedure and the reason remains unknown; this doesn't affect the therapy, which is focused on pain relief or nerve regeneration. As there is damage to the nerve, there are two types of pain: one that is spontaneously present, and one that is provoked by otherwise painless activities. This is characteristic of any type of neuralgia. There is also some genetic predisposition for the perception of neuropathic pain, because not everyone with nerve damage will experience pain. This depends on some proteins that are made under the regulation of genes, and this may be a link between the level of pain sensitivity and perception among individuals. Not everyone has the same pain threshold. That is why it is important to think about each person's individuality, in the anatomical and pathophysiological senses.

In many cases, a headache may appear to be caused by some problems in the neck. This could be a secondary type of headache, named cervicogenic headache, but actually, since nerves that exit the spinal cord spread their branches from the neck upwards to the head, it can be noted that these structures are closely connected. This can be applied to the neuralgia that appears at the back of the head: suboccipital and occipital neuralgia. Dysfunction or disposition of the vertebra, ligaments, or muscles of the neck may compress the nerves, thus inducing the headache.

The mechanism of facial neuralgias is similar, only located on the face, but it is also linked to the place where the nerves of the face originate from and the pathway that goes a long way to the area of innervation. The trigeminal nerve is responsible for sensation of the skin of the face. It originates from the brain stem and its pathway goes through the middle of the skull, where it meets various important organs and parts of the brain. When it is damaged, a person feels sensations, including pain, in one part of the face: upper, middle, or lower (most people feel pain in the lower part), which is usually placed on one side. Pain comes and vanishes suddenly. The pain is often referred to as *tic douloureux* or painful tic. Pain is triggered by various otherwise painless activities such as brushing teeth, touching the face, chewing, or speaking. With time, pain becomes more severe with time. It is difficult to treat, and some say that is the severest pain of all, almost like a cluster headache.

Other neuralgias appear when a nerve is damaged by infection or injury, or compressed by a blood vessel, muscle, or tumor. Glossopharyngeal, supraorbital, infraorbital, and occipital nerves induce pain in the area they innervate. Glossopharyngeal neuralgia is a rare condition and is more often linked to older age. The pain is located at the base of the tongue, in the throat, and is provoked by chewing and speaking. Supra- and infra-orbital nerves surround the eye cavity and are responsible for sensitivity of the eye and eyelid. When they are affected, there is an abnormality with pain sensation and increased perception in the area under or above the eye, with eye symptoms.

Occipital nerves are damaged in occipital neuralgia (C2 neuralgia). They originate in a place where there is great pressure from surrounding structures because of how a man's head is positioned during work or even at times when relaxing and resting. Any part of the body where there is a transition between two other large parts becomes sensitive. This is characteristic of joints; for example, the elbow and knee. These are the places where blood vessels are located on the surface and exposed to outer stimuli and injuries. The pain is located in the back of the head and is one-sided or, rarely, it appears on both sides. It is associated often with some other symptoms and problems with sensation. The pain is sharp and stabbing and it lasts for a couple of minutes per episode with high severity. The skin above the occipital nerve is sensitive and tender to touch. The neuralgias will be further discussed later. Their treatment is complex but usually involves antidepressants, anticonvulsants and physical therapy. (7)

Chapter 2. Neuralgia

Nerves may be either somatosensory or motoric. Motoric nerves are responsible for movement of the muscles. Somatosensory nerves have many functions, mainly the sensitive function, and they sometimes include autonomic nerve fibers. The autonomic nervous system is responsible for the involuntary function of the organs. For example, trigeminal nerve is a thick nerve that carries somatic fibers for sensations on the surface of the skin and, along the way, its branches receive special fibers that regulate the function of lachrymal gland, which is the gland that produces tears. This is important for people who experience pain in the face with watery eye.

Somatosensory nerves are responsible for sending out signals from the skin, subcutaneous tissue, organs, muscles, tendons, and joints. They send signals to the brain about changes in temperature, stretching, tension, pressure, or pain. Peripheral nerves receive stimuli from receptors on previously numbered tissues and send them to the spinal cord and to the brain. If there is damage to the tissue, a signal is sent within milliseconds as information about the damage.

Neuralgia (Greek *neuron*, which means nerve and *algos*, which means pain) is the type of pain that comes from nerves themselves with changed functions and thus the perception of pain may be greater than with any other type of pain. Another name for neuralgia is neuropathic pain. This pain originates solely from damage to the nerve and not necessarily to the tissue. A damaged nerve sends false signals to the brain, because its function is damaged as well. Pain may appear as stabbing or burning, with numbness and tingling. Also, the pain may be dull or sharp and may appear suddenly. It is specific for this type of pain to be triggered and provoked by minimal stimuli, touch or simple, otherwise non-painful activities, such as touching the skin, combing the hair, etc. This happens because of increased sensitivity of the nerve.

Neuralgia isn't a short-lasting type of pain that sends an alarm about damage to the tissue, which is called nocioceptive pain, but rather just pain signals that arise from even the slightest changes in function to the nerve. Because of that, it is called neuropathic pain. Nocioceptive pain brings the information to the brain about the damage if the nerves are preserved. If the nerves are destroyed, a person may experience no pain after injury or a phenomenon which is called "phantom" pain. This is characteristic with leg amputation. Along with any other structure of the leg, nerves are removed. However, after a while the person develops sharp or dull pain that is often resistant to treatment. People often describe it as a pain in the foot, like it is actually there, and injured.

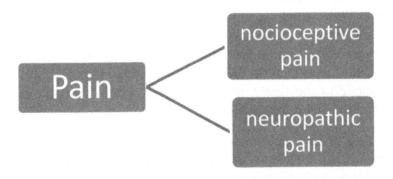

Neuropathic pain may be an individual condition or a consequence of a generalized illness; for example, diabetes mellitus. In diabetes mellitus, nerves are affected by a high level of glucose in the blood, which interferes with normal circulation. In diabetic neuropathy, blood vessels that supply the nerves (they too need nutrition) become damaged and send out false sensations of burning, tenderness, or stabbing pain. Typically, it appears in the legs, neck and face. Other than diabetic causes, there are neuralgias of face. The most common types of neuralgia are trigeminal neuralgia, occipital neuralgia, postherpetic neuralgia (a nerve infected with herpes zoster becomes sensitive even weeks and months after the infection), sciatic nerve pain (compression on the sciatic nerve and pain in the back and leg), intercostal neuralgia (nerves of rib cage have been compressed and induce pain in outer chest wall), and others. Facial and occipital neuralgia are among the most often diagnosed neuralgias. Neuralgia may become a permanent symptom and is sometimes even refractory to treatment.

As neuralgia becomes chronic, the person develops problems in his/her professional and personal life because of the pain and its consequences: fatigue, depression, loss of activity, worry, anxiety, nervousness, etc. It is widely known that the psychological state greatly influences the perception of pain. The stress and frustration arise from the pain, thus creating even other symptoms, an increase in the pain and more stress, anxiety and hopelessness. It is a closed circle that repeats.

Causes of neuralgia are:

- Infections (shingles-herpes zoster, syphilis, infection in the close surrounding of the nerve, leprosy, Lyme disease, Clostridium botulinum, HIV, EBV, CMV, West Nile virus, and some parasites, such as *Trypanosoma* from insect bites) can contribute to headaches by directly affecting the nerves or triggering the immune response that destroys nerves; they are usually easily treatable and preventable, but neuropathy may also develop as an adverse effect of antibacterial/antiviral therapy.
- Compression from surrounding tissue or swelling, tumor, blood vessels, tendons, or discs between vertebrae; holding the body in an uncomfortable, unchanging position may also compress the nerves; Some nerves are directly exposed to pressure from outside and structures inside that surround the nerve; symptoms include pain, tingling, numbness, pins and needles, weakness.
- Injury with swelling or direct compression on the nerve has similar mechanisms; injury is always an emergency

condition, while other causes above are only temporary and do not require medical assistance.

- Multiple sclerosis is a chronic illness where there is a complex mechanism of nerve damage and the most common pain is neuropathic pain; outer layers of the nerve are damaged, but there is also an inflammation of the nerve; one of the neuralgias is often present and that is trigeminal neuralgia; Lhermitte's sign is the pain in people with MS that develops suddenly and goes from back of the head, over the spine and to the arms and legs.
- Diabetes mellitus, metabolic liver diseases, low function of thyroid gland; diabetic neuropathic pain has been already mentioned and is maybe one of the most common neuropathic pains; lowered function of thyroid gland, hypothyroidism, induces neuropathic pain by keeping fluids and making the tissues swollen, and they might compress the nerves.
- Porphyria (blood disorder) is a rare chronic illness that includes abnormalities of the metabolic enzymes and thus leads to changed function in many organs.
- Chemical irritation may appear after injection or in other ways and is a consequence of a direct toxic effect on a nerve. Substances that might cause this even include some medications, anesthetics, but also some gas substances. This is very similar to multiple chemical sensitivity, a condition that is still a mystery. Namely, these people tend to have headaches after inhaling some substance, such as petroleum, for example. These, however, don't have a direct effect on the nerves as injection has.
- Chronic kidney disease may be the reason for headaches because of the rise of toxins that are not being excreted from the organism or some other unknown mechanism.
- Some medications (cisplatin, vincristine, paclitaxel for chemotherapy; antiretroviral therapy and anti-HIV medications; medications for high blood pressure)
- Alcohol use and B vitamin deficiency

- Surgery (sinus surgery, extraction of a tumor, surgery after trauma) can bring direct physical injury to the nerve.
- Unidentified/unknown cause. (8)

Damage to the nerves may be individual (mononeuropathy) or may include several nerves (polyneuropathy). The type of nerve injury depends on how much the nerve has been damaged. A nerve consists of two parts: its body with branches and the long branch, which connects with other nerves. This branch is an axon whose outer layers provide protection and integrity. The layer itself has the power to regenerate after injury, but the nerve cell doesn't. Depending on the depth and surface of the affected nerve damage to the peripheral nerves may be in form of:

- Neuropraxia (nerve is physically intact but its function is damaged; the injury is mild and with good prognosis for regeneration)
- Axonotmesis (the communicative branch, or axon, is damaged, which provides limited potential for regeneration)
- Neurotmesis (complete section of the nerve; the only way to connect the parts of the nerve is surgically).

In neuropraxia and axonotmesis, there is a possibility of spontaneous regeneration by the protective Schwann cells around nerve fibers. Occipital neuralgia is most likely caused by neuropraxia. As the nerve regenerates and heals, immunologic response may create a permanent structure called a neuroma that may be complicated treat. Therefore, it is important to evaluate the state of nerves and the possibility of surgical treatment. Some surgical treatments that include cutting the nerves also as a consequence develop neuromas. Fortunately, newer methods avoid this occurrence.

A person who complains of pain in any part of head or face must first receive the usual diagnostic assessment of surrounding organs and tissue (sinuses, ears, teeth, nose with tumor, inflammation, etc.) and then, if the pain stays unexplained and no structural cause is noted, neuralgia can be accepted as a possible cause of the pain.

Head neuralgias

In the head and face there are so many muscles and tendons that need to be innervated and controlled; that is why there are so many nerves in the head and face, and maybe that is why neuralgias are commonly manifested on the face. Also, there are some tight passages between bones and tendons or muscles, through which the nerves pass. This is where the nerve may be entrapped and become damaged. With damage, there is a change in function due to increased sensitivity to stimuli. This pain is described as very severe and disturbs a person greatly, changing the mood and behavior because of the pain and associated symptoms. However, the condition carries good prognostic factors and response to treatment.

There is a form of neuralgia from which occipital neuralgia should be distinguished. These neuralgias are located in different parts of the head, but still, as occipital neuralgia progresses, pain may spread to one side or the other.

Trigeminal neuralgia

Trigeminal neuralgia (*tic douloureux*) is a chronic type of pain that appears in trigeminal nerve, the fifth cranial nerve, which brings sensation to the face. The trigeminal nerve begins at the brain stem, spreads through the middle of the skull and then has three branches: ophthalmic, maxillary and mandibular, each for one-third of the face, the upper, middle, and lower parts. In trigeminal neuralgia, there is damage to one branch (usually) or more and an abnormal sensation in certain parts of the face, depending on the area and affected nerve that innervates it. Trigeminal neuralgia is the most common neuralgia located on the head.

The ophthalmic nerve supplies the area of scalp, forehead, and above the eye. The maxillary nerve covers the middle of the face:

cheeks, upper lip, upper jaw, and teeth and gums in the upper jaw. The mandibular nerve innervates the lower part of the face: the lower jaw, the teeth and gums there, and the bottom lip. Usually, one side is affected in trigeminal neuralgia, or the sides switch periodically.

This happens most commonly to persons around the age of 50. There are two types of trigeminal neuralgia, type 1 and 2. Type 1, a classical trigeminal neuralgia, is a disorder that appears more frequently. In classical trigeminal neuralgia, pain is sudden and sharp, electric shock-like. It lasts for couple of seconds or minutes. Sometimes people with multiple sclerosis (MS) also have trigeminal neuralgia. Pain appears around teeth, mouth, nose, or cheek. Type 1 is more severe than type 2. Type 2, which is sometimes called atypical or symptomatic trigeminal neuralgia, actually represents less severe symptoms, and both may appear in the same person. In type 2, pain is almost always present, dull and stabbing, with lower intensity than in type 1. The cause in most cases remains unknown. The most common cause is compression of the surrounding blood vessel and the most common place for nerve compression is the place where the nerve exits the brain stem. Other structures that might compress the nerve are tumors or inflamed and swollen tissue after infection, injury, or surgery. Direct compression provokes damage to the outer layers of the nerve, which interrupts transmission of signals. Any damage to the layer around the nerve may be followed with symptoms, since it too is responsible for sending signals for sensation and with damage comes the abnormal nerve response with numbness, tingling, and pain. Even though there must be damage to the nerve in order for neuralgia to appear, the nerve is usually visually intact, so maybe there are some mild changes and functional disorder in the nerve.

Symptoms are recurrent, appearing suddenly as an ''electric shock,'' followed by long-lasting dull pain. Bouts of pain may appear several times a day, but rarely during the night. Shocking pain lasts for a short while and diminishes within seconds, while some discomfort and less severe pain stay longer. Some people don't even have any painful sensation between the bouts. Also, it is characteristic for pain not to appear at night. Pain is triggered by otherwise painless activities, such as touching the skin, chewing, speaking, a cool breeze, or cold food and drinks. That is why people with trigeminal neuralgia may develop eating disorders and different social behavior, with difficulties and fear of speaking, which can easily be followed with depression. This is how multiple sclerosis is connected, since in MS the myelin layer is damaged, i.e., demyelination occurs.

Diagnosis is usually reached after other illnesses have been excluded and after symptomatology and diagnostic tests confirm that the condition corresponds with trigeminal neuralgia. In order to exclude some serious illnesses, a person is advised to undergo MRI diagnostic assessment.

Treatment includes antidepressants and antiepileptics (anticonvulsives such as carbamazepine and oxcarbazepine), that are also medications for neuropathic pain. Commonly used analgesics, NSAIDs and opioid, morphine-based analgesics do not help in neuralgias. Other choices for treatment are: topiramate, gabapentin, pregabalin, clonazepam, phenytoin, lamotrigine, and valproic acid, muscle relaxants, and surgery. (9)

Supraorbital and infraorbital neuralgia are sometimes considered subtypes of trigeminal neuralgia, since they are the branches from maxillary and ophthalmic branches.

Supraorbital neuralgia (SON)

Supraorbital neuralgia is a rare disorder. This neuralgia affects the supraorbital nerve, which is responsible for innervation of the area above the eye and the eyebrow and forehead from each side. The cause may be trauma, infection, compression, or inflammation, or it may remain unknown. Swimmers who wear goggles, for example, sometimes develop headaches in the area of the eye, forehead, and scalp after wearing them too tight. Pain is usually one-sided and it can be triggered by otherwise painless activities such as touching or combing the hair or touching the skin. Pain is chronic, and appears in form of intermittent bouts and reliefs. Other than pain, supraorbital neuralgia may include numbness or tingling or other types of abnormal sensation of the forehead.

Diagnosis is given after the exclusion of any other condition, with symptoms that correspond to neuropathy of supraorbital nerve. Sometimes a person needs an MRI or CT scan just to be sure that the cause isn't structural. Therapy includes medication (antidepressants and anticonvulsants), nerve blocks (which are also used to prove the diagnosis of supraorbital neuralgia), and sometimes surgery. (10)

Infraorbital neuralgia (ION)

Similar to supraorbital neuralgia, infraorbital appears because of damage to the infraorbital nerve that innervates the area beneath the eye and the cheeks. Pain is also one-sided. Possible causes are infections, trauma, or surgery on the maxillary sinus, or the cause may remain unknown. It may also be provoked by some otherwise painless actions. Diagnosis is based on nerve blocks, CT, MRI. Treatment is similar to supraorbital neuralgia.

Neuropathic facial pain

This neuralgia isn't as typical as others, but it has symptoms that may resemble trigeminal neuralgia. The pathophysiology is different and the nerve may or may not be injured or damaged. It is also referred to as atypical facial pain or persistent idiopathic facial pain (PIFP). In the process of development, any factors may be included: infective, inflammatory, traumatic, tumors, etc. They affect the trigeminal nerve. It may appear as very similar to trigeminal neuralgia but the affected area isn't the same as in trigeminal neuralgia; rather, it spreads without any specific rule. The pain usually lasts for hours. It may last the whole day with periods of painlessness. The pain is usually on both sides of the face. This condition is suggested when all the other explanations do not fit the condition better. Besides the causes such as compression of the nerve and similar organic problems, it also has some psychological influences in pathophysiology. It is difficult distinguishing which nerve is affected when symptoms do not correspond with any area of innervations. The differences and boundaries between trigeminal neuralgia and PIFP remain unstable. In PIFP, there is no triggered response to otherwise painless activities.

Diagnosis is focused on excluding other, more likely explanations. Treatment is usually less successful and includes antidepressants, anticonvulsives, and cognitive behavioral treatment.

Glossopharyngeal Neuralgia (GPN)

Glossopharyngeal nerve is the ninth cranial nerve, which is responsible for sensations in the mouth, tongue, tonsils, and throat and brings sensation of smell to the brain. It also has a role in regulation of blood pressure, heartbeat, frequency of breathing, vomiting, and swallowing, although the nervus vagus has the key role in these functions. These functions are provided with fibers of the autonomic nervous system. Glossopharyngeal neuralgia is pain that appears in the throat, tongue, and tonsils and spreads to the ear, so it may look like a respiratory infection and an ear infection. For a long time it may appear so and the real cause remains hidden. Glossopharyngeal nerve may be either compressed by a blood vessel, a tumor, or inflammatory and infectious masses in tonsils and throat, or in Eagle's syndrome by abnormally long styloid process from the temporal bone. In many cases, the cause remains unexplained. It appears more frequently in men older than 40. It is a condition with a good prognosis and successful treatment.

The pain is often described as very severe. Bouts of pain may occur many times a day with pauses and painless periods and with great effect on the person's quality of life. It can be triggered by chewing, speaking, coughing, yawning, or sneezing. This is evidently creating many problems in everyday life. The pain is usually present on one side, and lasts about 30 seconds. Pain is often shock-like, sharp, and sudden, located deep in the throat. Even though attacks come and go, the periods with pain may bring pain with higher intensity that lasts even longer than before. Other than pain, a person may experience problems with hearing, which might disturb him/her, and also some vegetative symptoms such as nausea, vomiting, buzzing in the ears, problems with movement, dizziness, and loss of consciousness may worsen the clinical picture. In this neuralgia and nerve damage there could be some complications because of its regulation of vital functions. Therefore, arrhythmias, loss of consciousness, or convulsions may appear.

Glossopharyngeal neuralgia is a rare disorder and it is somewhat more frequently diagnosed in women, for unknown reasons. Diagnosis is approved with a clinical exam and some advanced diagnostic procedures (CT, MRI) that need to exclude causes such as tumors. As with trigeminal neuralgia, treatment is based on antidepressants and anticonvulsants (antiepileptics) that are used for treatment of neuropathic pain, nerve blocks and surgical treatment. (11)

Occipital neuralgia (ON)

Occipital neuralgia or C2 or Arnold's neuralgia is a subject of this book, with more information that follows. It is a neuropathic pain that originates from the occipital nerves, most commonly the greater and lesser occipital nerves. They are either compressed with muscles, blood vessels, inflammation of the tissue, or trauma, and that induces pain that rises from the neck to the top of the scalp. It can also cause sensitivity to light and hypersensitivity to painful and painless activities. It is very difficult to distinguish it from a migraine and some other neuralgias, since it is a much rarer condition than them. The modern lifestyle, with sitting in uncomfortable positions, increases the prevalence of this condition.

Chapter 3. Occipital nerves anatomy

Occipital neuralgia was first described in 1821 and was originally named Arnold's neuralgia after Dr. Arnold, a famous neurologist. It isn't a common condition, but many people discover symptoms and pain in the back of the head and neck and it occurs more than we tend to admit. In order to understand the mechanism by which occipital neuralgia develops, we need to take a look at how the nerves are placed and how they can become damaged. Occipital nerves are placed on a very sensitive area of the head, where large muscles attach to the bones and where there is a large pressure from the head, which is heavy. The muscles around the bones of head and neck need to be strong to hold the head in position and move it in various directions. After many years of overuse, these strong muscles become exhausted and "damaged." As they become damaged, they suffer inflammation with swelling, stiffness, and rigid movement. The inflammatory cells on site are responsible for healing. Thus the possibility of direct compression to the nerves from the uncomfortable, exhausting positions during working days that usually include sitting with head placed straight forward or bent down, at the desk, in front of computers or work at a machine.

The anatomy of these structures follows. We need to begin from the spinal cord, where the occipital nerves originate. The spinal cord is placed in a tight bone structure, the vertebral column. The complex anatomy of the neck begins in the junction between the vertebral column's neck part and the bones of the back of the head. This junction is especially a vulnerable place that is predisposed for damage to the sensitive structures.

Vertebral column

The vertebral column (spine) is a strong, flexible bone structure that distends from the back of the head and occipital bone and goes all the way to the back of the pelvis. It is built from vertebrae, irregularly shaped bones that are divided into segments according to the region and the function they provide: cervical-C (neck), thoracic-Th (rib cage), lumbar-L (lower back), sacral-S (back wall of the pelvis), and the coccygeal bone. Bodies of vertebrae are becoming larger going from the neck, to the chest, and the largest ones are located on the lower back, and these vertebrae are the largest because of the enormous pressure and weight they carry. Below the lumbar segment, the vertebrae become smaller again, only to end in a tail-like structure in the pelvis. Inside the vertebral column, there is a spinal canal that is completely surrounded and in which the spinal cord lies protected. Its function is to protect the spinal cord but it also provides the posture and stability of upright position. From the spinal cord, roots exit that are responsible for innervation of the surrounding and distant structures.

The vertebral bones are connected with each other by various ligaments, joint capsules, and muscles and the bodies of the bones are vertically connected by intervertebral discs that form a cushion between them. The discs may become damaged and begin to change position and exit from the tight space between the vertebra, thus compressing the surrounding nerves that exit from the spinal cord. According to some theories, the liquid from the disc may cause chemical irritation to the surrounding nerves. The cervical segment of the spine may also degenerate with age and the vertebrae become fused and form a bamboo stick-like structure. This may also induce pain in the neck when the head is bent down. Ligaments may become calcified, elongated, or pinched as they too pass through tight spaces in bones. These ligaments may in different mechanisms be responsible for incarceration of the occipital nerves (atlanto-axial joint). The first vertebra is called the atlas (in Greek mythology, Atlas was a titan who was punished and ordered to hold the Earth on his shoulders). The atlas is joined with occipital bone of the skull. Misalignment of the atlas may be the cause of neck pain, and it develops from abnormal positions assumed during working days or improper long-lasting positions during rest time, etc. If the atlas is not in its right place, it may begin to compress the arteries and nerves, inducing pain. The axis is the second vertebra and is connected to the atlas with a pointy part that provides rotation movements of the head. As the atlas becomes misaligned, it leads to misalignment of other vertebrae, as well. Huge trauma and injuries to these vertebrae may also induce pain in the back of the head and neck (whiplash injury). It is also important to mention that the spinal nerve roots exit from the spinal cord between the occipital bone and the atlas (C1), between the atlas and the axis (C2), and between the axis and the third cervical vertebra (C3). Degeneration of C1 and C2 vertebrae, specifically, may be responsible for occipital neuralgia.

Occipital bone and occipitalis muscle

The occipital bone is a flat bone located at the back of the head; it covers the occipital lobe of the brain and the small brain (*lat. cerebellum*). Over the occipital bone lies the dense layer of fibrous tissue, which is stretched over the top of the head and then connects with muscles of the front and back. This firm and strong mass of fibrous tissue is called *galea aponeurotica* and plays the role of a tendon for the large muscles of the head. The occipitalis muscle lies on the surface of the occipital bone. It is considered to be part of the occipitofrontalis muscle, which stretches from the forehead to the neck-head junction. The occipitalis muscle can cause occipital pain, for example, after keeping the eyebrows raised for too long or because of tension. This muscle lies under the greater occipital nerve and its branches, but its role in occipital neuralgia isn't significant.

Spinal cord

The spinal cord is a part of the central nervous system, which also includes the whole brain and brainstem. The spinal cord distends from the brain stem in the back of the head to the area where lumbar and sacral vertebrae meet at the lower back. Along its way through the spine, the spinal cord has branches for innervations of skin, muscles, and organs for the various regions. Actually, from the spinal cord on both sides two roots arise, for the left and right sides. The roots are then divided into two branches that go to the front and back, and give rise to nerves as well, but then they unite again and form a *spinal nerve* that again divides into front and back branches. The rear branch of each root contains a ganglion, which is an important spot for surgical intervention in treatment of pain. Spinal nerves have sensory and motoric functions, i.e., for muscles and autonomic fibers inside them. There are 31 pairs, left and right, that arise from the spinal cord.

In occipital neuralgia, the occipital nerves are important for us; they arise from C2 and C3 spinal nerves. There is also another nerve structure called the cervical plexus, which is built from front branches of the spinal nerves from C1 to C4 in the neck and is responsible for innervation of the neck including skin and muscles.

The dorsal (back) branch of C2, the cervical part of spinal cord, second segment, builds the greater occipital nerve and it arises more to the midline from lesser occipital nerve, which are both important in development of occipital neuralgia. The dorsal branch of C3 builds the third occipital nerve.

Cervical plexus

The cervical plexus (Figure 1) is built from cervical spinal nerves, the front (ventral) branches from C1 to C4, and they combine with each other. This builds many nerves. The branches are: Phrenic nerve (for innervation of diaphragm), nerves for innervations of muscles on the front of the neck and help with speech and swallowing, some nerves for innervations of the lateral part of the neck, but also sensory nerves: the lesser occipital nerve, greater auricular, transverse cervical, and some supraclavicular nerves. From it also arises the lesser occipital nerve, which is important for the pathology of occipital neuralgia, but less often than the greater occipital nerve. The cervical plexus may be damaged by car accidents, surgeries in the close area, sports injuries, and other cause. Each of these injuries may harm any branch whose fibers are included in the lesser occipital nerve, and this may change the function of the nerve from the proximal to the distal part. The pain that appears is located in different areas of the head, neck, and arms, depending on the nerve that was pinched or damaged.

Occipital nerves

There are three occipital nerves: The greater occipital nerve, the lesser occipital nerve and the third occipital nerve. Another nerve that can be responsible for occipital neuralgia is the suboccipital nerve, but here it will only be mentioned because of its lesser significance. They rise from the spinal cord upward to the top of the head. The area they spread on is between the midline that divides two sides, left and right, and the ear lobe, and on the upper side they cover the surface of the scalp on the top of the head. The area they innervate might be deeper than just the muscles and skin, because the pain when the nerves are affected spreads deep into the eye on the same side. The closest to the ear is the lesser occipital nerve, the greater is in the middle, and the third lies almost in the midline. The suboccipital nerve exits the spinal cord between the atlas and occipital bone and is a branch of the C1 nerve. It lies in suboccipital triangle.

1. *The greater occipital nerve* (Figure 2) arises from the second cervical nerve C2 from the spinal cord and exits between the atlas and the axis, the first and second neck vertebrae. It begins on the rear branch of spinal nerve C2. Probably the illness itself got the name after the origin of this nerve, as it is the most responsible of all occipital nerves. Its function involves sensations in the back of the head and scalp. It is linked to migraines and other types of headaches, including occipital neuralgia. This nerve is damaged in most of the people who also have neck problems, and it is indeed the typical occipital neuralgia. Sensations arise from the neck and back of the head to the top of the head and may also spread to the eye. In 45% of people, the greater occipital nerve passes through the trapezius muscle, a large muscle in the back of the neck. This could be the way occipital neuralgia develops: The

muscle compresses the nerve and thus pain is induced. The greater occipital nerve passes beneath inferior obliquus capitis muscle and beneath the suboccipital triangle built from the obliquus capitis superior, and the inferior and rectus capitis posterior major. These three muscles build a triangle. In this triangle of strong muscles in the neck area, a nerve may become entrapped when muscles are used inappropriately and excessively. For example, when a person holds the head either to the side, up, or down for a long time, it may require large amounts of energy for the muscle to sustain that position. As a result of the excessive use, they become inflamed, swollen, and very tender to touch. As they increase their volume, they may compress surrounding structures including the occipital nerves, especially in as tight a structure as the suboccipital triangle. Contents of the suboccipital triangle are: branches of vertebral artery (that supplies the back part of the brain), the suboccipital venous plexus, and the suboccipital nerve from C1. The occipital nerves are positioned close to the suboccipital triangle and that is how they are affected, especially the greater occipital nerve. After the triangle, the greater occipital nerve reaches the great trapezius muscle, which is the largest muscle of the back of the neck, covering all of the other smaller muscles of the back of the neck. The nerve goes through a small a canal in the muscle. If we consider how much pressure is laid on that muscle with every movement not only of the neck but also of the face and arms, we can easily imagine that this muscle must be very strong, and sometimes it isn't strong enough for the great tension it endures. It can too easily be inflamed, which compress the greater occipital nerve. After the trapezius muscle, the greater occipital nerve goes upwards and to the scalp over the surface of the occipital muscle and bone. It goes to the front, where it ends with smaller branches, forming a tree-like structure. It is responsible for dissemination of the pain from the back of the head all the way to the scalp. In addition to muscles, nerves can be affected by injuries and systemic illnesses, and with tumors or blood vessels that compress the nerve.

2. ***The lesser (small) occipital nerve*** arises from C2 and C3 spinal nerves in the cervical plexus. The greater and lesser occipital nerves are the most significant in the pathophysiology of occipital pain. The lesser occipital nerve innervates the area behind the earlobe and the side part of the scalp. That is why the symptoms of affected nerves are abnormal skin sensations and pain. It exits the cervical part of spinal cord within the cervical plexus, as a combined, united branch, and goes over the back border of the great muscle sternocleidomastoideus. This muscle goes from the upper border of the chest to the back of the ear and the bone part of the skull called the mastoid. With compression of the sternocleidomastoideus, the lesser occipital nerve changes its function. After it passes behind the ear, it goes upwards and communicates with other nerves of the scalp, as well. In damage to the lesser occipital nerve, a person may experience pain in the side of the head.

3. ***The third occipital nerve*** and suboccipital nerve are less significant in the pathophysiology of occipital neuralgia, but will be mentioned anyway. The third, or least occipital nerve, arises from C2 and C3. It is responsible for innervation of the back of the skull. This nerve is often injured in car accidents (whiplash injury). It lies beneath the trapezius muscle, and is sometimes compressed with it when it is overused and swollen. It ends at the lower parts of the back of the neck. Osteoarthritis (degeneration that comes with age or long-term improper use of the neck) of the C2-3 side facet joint of cervical spine may also induce headaches because of the effect on the third occipital nerve that innervates this joint. This nerve innervates the skin above this region, so the trigger points for pain are located in the small area of skin above the joint in the neck. (12) (13)

4. ***Suboccipital nerve*** arises from the C1, the first cervical spinal nerve. C1 exits between the occipital bone and the

atlas, so basically the head lies on it. It goes through the suboccipital triangle, which is built from the previously mentioned structures, muscles. This spot is vulnerable, along with the greater occipital nerve. Along with nerve goes the occipital artery, which can also have some role in the pathology of this nerve when they interweave. (14)

The Cervical Plexus

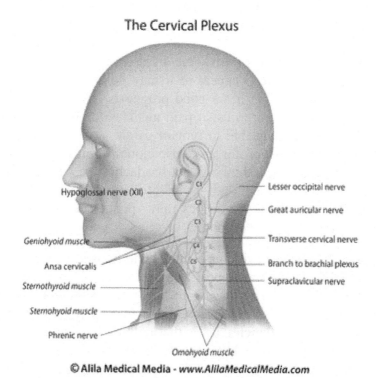

© Alila Medical Media - www.AlilaMedicalMedia.com

Figure 1 Innervation of the head from the cervical branches from spinal cord – cervical plexus. Front branches of spinal nerve unite to form individual nerves for certain area of the back of the head.

Chapter 4. Occipital headaches and pain in the back of the head

Occipital pain is pain in the back of the head. It can bring a lot of discomfort, because of the sensitivity of area. The pain may induce fear and worry because it can easily bring the feeling as if something grabbed the back of the head, and disabled movement. The reasons for the pain that appears suddenly or gradually may vary. They could be the warning signs of upcoming complications from some diseases such as tumors, high blood pressure, or sleep apnea, or it may be a benign pain that needs to be treated, but has a good prognosis. This pain may be disturbing and resistant to usual pain medication and good sleep. It isn't always manageable to remain painless and it is good to visit the doctor's office for any suspicions. Many people don't report their headaches, thinking that headaches are very common in human population and that it will resolve itself, but that is not necessarily true. Some headaches may spontaneously disappear but return after a couple of months or years.

The table that follows will number the conditions in which pain in the back of the head may appear as a symptom. When all of them are excluded, we can talk about occipital neuralgia and its management. A lot of these conditions may also be causes of occipital neuralgia, which tells us that nothing is black and white in medicine and health. The illnesses combine with each other. Some of them are severe and some are benign and only temporary.

Illness	Description
Neck spine and ligament degeneration	Any degeneration to the joint components is followed by slipping off the whole structure and losing the stability, with possible compression to the surrounding nerves and arteries. Previous injuries and

	older age are the precipitating factors that accelerate the process of degeneration of the cartilage which becomes vulnerable with lack of water in it.
Brain tumors	Primary and secondary (metastatic) tumors in the back of the head may induce pain, but sometimes the diagnosis is determined earlier or with the appearance of other symptoms that indicate destruction of the nerves.
Compression of the nerves, radiculopathy	Surrounding tissues and organs may push and press the nerves, thus affecting their function. A nerve root can become compressed by bone and fibrous tissue, and nerves in the area of the neck and head are surrounded with arteries that may cross over them and compress them, interfering with their function.
Rheumatoid arthritis	This is a chronic illness that affects small joints of the hands but also joints of the neck. The mechanism is autoimmune. The affected joint is atlanto-axial, with irritation to the spinal nerve and pain in the back of the head.
Tension, cluster, migraine headaches	Even though these headaches have typical zones of pain that do not usually appear at the back of the head, they are worth mentioning, for the mixed etiology and possible effect on the structures at the back of the head. There is a condition in which migraine and occipital neuralgia exist as a conjoined illness.
Ice pick headache	This headache is described as a sharp pain, as if a needle or ice pick is being stabbed into the head. The pain may be located in any part of the head, including the back of the head.

Ice cream headache	Brain-freeze, as it is commonly called, is the consequence of quickly drinking or eating cold food such as ice cream or cold drinks. The pain is usually temporary and located at the side or the back of the head.
Dialysis headache	Dialysis is a treatment of chronic kidney failure and it too may be the reason for sudden appearance of headaches. They appear because of the large amounts of water and electrolytes that suddenly enter the blood stream, disrupting the inner electrolyte and fluid balance.
Orgasmic headache	Headaches may appear in any phase of sexual intercourse and are a consequence of constriction of blood vessels.
Increased intracranial pressure	Tumors, bleeding, blockages, and injuries may contribute to an increase of pressure in the head, where free space is already small. This can be manifested by headaches, but very often with other symptoms, as well. Pain appears in the back of the head when the process is in that part of the head.
Inflammation of arteries (temporal arteritis)	Temporal arteritis spreads over the side of the head and, when it is inflamed, it causes pulsating pain along its course on the side of the head. The pain may spread to the rear side as well.
Bleeding in the brain and meninges	Bleeding from unknown reasons, such as rupture of the artery malformation, aneurysm, or as a consequence of illness.
Dissection of the arteries at the back of the head (vertebral arteries)	Vertebral arteries are essentially two arteries in the back of the neck, providing the blood supply to the structures of the brain. Dissection happens rarely in vertebral arteries, but is an important cause of a stroke.

Sleep apnea	Condition with problems of breathing overnight, when a person has 100 episodes of non-breathing and then wakes each time after that. As a consequence, a person is sleepy during the day, and doesn't remember being awake. Headaches during the day appear specifically in the back of the head.
Parkinson's disease	Chronic illness with progressive movement problems and tremors, with headaches located in the back of the head as a consequence of changed posture and an illness in general.
Inflammation in the throat, retropharyngeal tendinitis	Inflammation deep in the throat, with pain in the back of the head and while swallowing and speaking.
Inflammation of the sinuses	Usually, pain from the affected sinus is located in the face or in the area deep behind the eyes. The pain may also spread to the back of the head as the infection progresses.
Shingles (herpes zoster)	Skin rash with blisters and pain at one specific area are characteristics of shingles, caused by the herpes zoster virus. When the virus infects the nerves at the back of the head, that is where the symptoms will appear. The virus stays in hibernation in nerve ganglions and, in situations where immunity is compromised, the virus acts again.
Swollen lymph nodes	As infection progresses, it affects the lymph nodes and they might become painfully enlarged and skin becomes reddish.
Meningitis	This infection of the outer layers of the brain can be the cause of the pain in the

	occipital area, depending on where the source of the infection is. Along with headache come other symptoms such as high fever, light sensitivity, nausea and vomiting, and a stiff neck.
Blood pressure	Even though it is common to experience pain in the side of the head, some people have pain at the back of the head. Some people have pain in this region and in the neck and then, after measuring the blood pressure, they notice that it is increased. These headaches are not, however, considered as signs of high blood pressure, which is asymptomatic in many people. Headaches appear only in people who are prone to develop headaches in general. (15)
Coughing and straining	Coughing, straining, and similar activities may increase pressure in abdomen but also in the head, which may provoke headaches.
Heart illness	Some people report that, when they suffered a heart attack, they felt pain in the chest but also in the back of the head. This is yet to be explained scientifically, for the mechanism is probably anxiety and straining or something entirely different.
Injuries to the muscles of the neck	Muscle that is injured is becoming inflamed and enlarged, sensitive to touch and movement. It can compress the nerves that are nearby.
Enormous heights	People who are not acclimated to low oxygen level and high atmospheric pressure may experience pain in the head and very rarely they feel pain at the back of the head.

Increased thyroid function	Headaches may appear as a symptom of increased function of thyroid gland, thyrotoxicosis, but it is always associated with other specific thyroid symptoms. (16)
Occipital neuralgia	Damage to the occipital nerves.

Occipital neuralgia. How many people have this type of headache?

Occipital neuralgia isn't precisely defined and criteria have not been decided upon. Trigeminal neuralgia is the most common neuralgia in the head, but it is very rare (4-5 in 100,000 people). Only 3.2 in 100,000 people have occipital neuralgia, according to the American Headache and Migraine Association. (17) Occipital neuralgia affects men and women equally, no matter what age they are. Some studies showed somewhat higher prevalence in women, but women are also more likely to visit a doctor's office to seek some advice. Often, people do not visit a doctor for the pain in the head, at least not until the pain is severe. That is why the statistics on this condition are incomplete.

There are reports that migraine affects the greater occipital nerve, which may indicate that there is a mixed etiology for a headache. This happens rarely and is referred to as a migraine involving the greater occipital nerve and the reason for this is the convergence of the pathways of the nerves affected in the migraine and occipital nerves. These patients have all of the symptoms of the migraine but also a pain in the back of the head. This may cause confusion between the two conditions (or all three). That is why it is hard to calculate the statistical prevalence of occipital headache. (18)

There are many structures along the occipital nerves, especially around the greater occipital nerve, that can press the nerve because of their position. Some scientists consider true occipital neuralgia to be the one where the cause isn't known and all of the other causes such as muscle entrapment or compression of a blood vessel, joint, bone, or ligament may be differently categorized, not as true occipital neuralgia. Some, however, consider this condition to be a large group of disorders with either unknown or known, structural cause. It is all about the symptom of pain in the head with its associated symptoms which require treatment for pain relief.

Etiology. How and why does occipital neuralgia develop?

We can divide causes of occipital neuralgia into two categories: primary, with unknown cause (most often), or secondary, structural, when there is some damage to the nerve or compression that changes the function of the nerve and induces pain. Primary occipital neuralgia is idiopathic, or with unknown causes, which doesn't deny all of the symptoms that a person has, but the headache doesn't correspond to any visible anatomical damage to the nerves or surrounding tissue in a way that it could explain the symptoms. Most of the people don't have visible structural changes that could indicate a clear damage to the nerves. Secondary occipital neuralgia can have one, or sometimes more than one possible cause for the development. These causes are:

Injury - Specifically, *Whiplash* injury is in many cases the cause for the headache at the back of the head. (19) The injury happens while driving, when a car suddenly stops, whether because of sudden braking or hitting an object. A person has fastened the seatbelt, but the head moves forward or backwards and during that rapid, sudden movement, structures of the neck may be injured, including the occipital nerves. That is why this type of injury is called whiplash, because a sudden movement of the neck may cause severe damage to the neck. Whiplash does not develop only in car accidents. For it to happen, the same mechanism of injury has to happen. Other types of injuries can also lead to pain in the back of the head, such as when a person is directly hit on the back of the head or has fallen on the back of the head.

Inflammation – Local inflammatory processes may cause tissue to swell, expand, and compress the nerves. During inflammatory processes, some substances are excreted from the tissue as a response to some agent that is compromising or damaging the tissue. These substances tend to alarm the cells from the blood stream. These cells are protectors and fight the agents and also facilitate healing. With them, a lot of fluid passes from the blood stream into the area of inflammation in order to dilute the microorganisms and facilitate the fight against them. This is typical for local infective inflammations that originate from the skin, subcutaneous tissue, bones, etc. Other than microorganisms, some other factors may stimuli the secretion of these substances. These can be the damage to the muscles and their swelling, irritation of the tissue, etc.

Swollen muscles are actually the most common reason for occipital neuralgia and they appear as a reaction to overuse. Muscles included in pathogenesis are the great muscles of the neck and back of the head: the trapezius, semispinalis capitis, and obliquus capitis inferior muscles (builds the previously mentioned suboccipital triangle). These muscles are very strong and their function is to hold the head and move it in various directions. If they get inflamed and swollen because of improper and excessive use, they will compress the occipital nerve and provoke the symptoms. It is important to know the pathway of the occipital nerves and their position over the muscles. These nerves pass across and close to the suboccipital triangle and the greater occipital nerve passes through a small hole in the trapezius muscle. These zones are especially vulnerable for development of pain in the neck and back of the head. The suboccipital triangle is located beneath the large trapezius muscle in the pit on both sides of the neck. In this tight space of muscles, artery, and nerves, any expansion of tissue complicates with compression on either artery or nerve.

Systemic disease and diabetes – Lupus is mentioned as one of the most frequent reasons for occipital neuropathy and neuralgia. The mechanism by which this happens is not well understood, but scientists have theories about antibodies and neurotoxins that are present in people with lupus. In other systemic autoimmune diseases, neurological complications appear rarely. (20) Other types of diseases, such as diabetes, involve nerves differently. In diabetes mellitus, nerves are damaged because the circulation is damaged by the high blood sugar level, which impairs the nourishment of nerves. However, some complex mechanisms may play a role in specific development of occipital neuralgia in people with diabetes and not just the blood vessel damage with high levels of sugar.

Osteoarthritis, degenerative cervical spine, gout – These problems may cause the cervical spine to take a different position, and thereby compress the occipital nerves. In osteoarthritis and degeneration of the cervical spine, bones of the vertebral column are losing their matrix and that can be considered as a part of the normal aging process. However, some are more predisposed to develop problems in the neck movement and pain in the back of the head. These people, during their work time throughout life, held the neck in uncomfortable positions, with the head down, which placed a great pressure on the muscles and bones of the neck. That is why changes in the neck will appear sooner in these people than in other people. This headache is referred to as cervicogenic. Nerve roots are close to the vertebrae and ligaments, so the compression may appear in larger areas of the neck and scalp. Gout is a chronic illness with deposition of crystals of uric acid in many areas in the body. The illness also affects bones and joints. Because of the crystals of uric acid, joints are swollen and painful, with decreased movement. This may lead to occipital neuralgia. All of these conditions may compress the occipital nerve or C2 spinal nerve on one side, thus provoking symptoms. Some spine developmental deformities may also be responsible for occipital neuralgia. The symptoms develop gradually, since the degeneration develops over many years.

Cervical disc disease is also a degenerative condition, in which the disc between two cervical vertebrae is swollen and slowly, over the years, changes its structure, escapes its normal position, and begins compressing the surrounding nerves, which can cause the symptoms. There is evidence of toxic effects of the liquid from disc on the nerves. Cervical disc disease also appears in people who overuse the neck or hold the head in an uncomfortable position for too long.

Blood vessels that have enlarged walls and that surround occipital nerves may be another reason for occipital neuralgia. Aneurysms are localized expansions of the artery walls. They are, however, rare in this region. Another possibility is that blood vessels are inflamed for various reasons (idiopathic, infective agents, autoimmune diseases). Abnormal position of the blood vessels, arteriovenous fistulas, and bleeding are some of the reason why a person might be experiencing occipital headache. When the artery interweaves with the nerve, the nerve may be compressed by a thick wall of the artery, and the nerve won't impair the blood supply. All of these vascular conditions are infrequent in the population. (21) (22)

Tumors, such as meningioma for example, may have their first symptom in the form of occipital headache. Meningiomas are benign tumors that grow from the cells of layers around the brain tissue, causing the intracranial pressure to rise and induce some symptoms depending on the area where they develop. If meningioma develops in the part where head and neck meet, close to the great opening in the skull, it will compress the nerves between C1 and C3. However, this happens rarely. (23)

Chapter 5. Occipital neuralgia symptoms

Occipital neuralgia is a typical neurological disorder with symptoms that appear the same as with any other damage to the nerves. When a nerve is pinched or compressed and its function is changed, a person develops symptoms such as tenderness, numbness, pain triggered by otherwise painless actions, including touching the skin, combing the hair, wiping, and other activities on the skin, along with pain that isn't triggered. The neuropathic pain is stabbing and sharp, usually sudden and it may appear as an electric shock, shock-like, but it can also appear as dull, throbbing, and continuous pain. Occipital neuralgia includes the following symptoms:

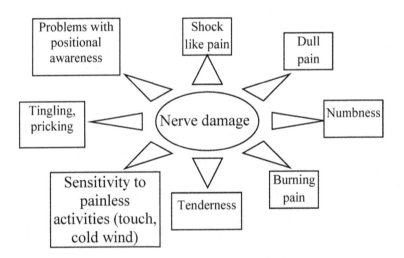

Allodynia is pain that is triggered by otherwise painless activities. It is a reaction to otherwise ordinary and painless actions that do not normally stimulate the pain receptors. These can be mild touch, heat, wind, cold, a pin-prick, pressure, and it is classified into categories according to those. It is specific for any neuralgia to be provoked with any contact with the nerve, along its way, or at the area of the skin innervated by that nerve. This happens because the nerve is damaged and the receptors become more sensitive to any other stimuli, which are otherwise harmless, in order to protect the tissue and promote healing. It isn't necessarily the sign of an illness but rather of some harm that threatens to damage the tissue and requires protective measures. It is often combined with hyperalgesia. Not all people will develop these symptoms. They appear in 20% of people with neuropathies. Allodynia means that pain comes from other stimuli (*allos*, Greek). (24)

Paresthesia appears from damage to the sensitive function of the nerve, which creates symptoms such as numbness, tingling, burning, or pricking, the damaged nerve sends out false signals, like there is burning of the skin or like real needles are pricking the skin. This tells us about changed functions. It is an abnormal sensation that can be temporary or long-term. The sensation happens even in ordinary situations which we have all encountered: after sleeping on arm or after hitting an elbow in the area where the nerve is exposed. This induces numbness and pricking, which is very uncomfortable. After the pressure on the nerve is removed, symptoms gradually fade away. Sometimes the pressure can't be removed physically, and indicates a neurological disorder. Paresthesia in occipital neuralgia brings similar symptoms.

The word *paresthesia* comes from *esthesia*, which is a capability of sensation, and *par-*, a prefix that describes abnormality of something. In the same way, anesthesia describes the inability to sensate, which happens intentionally during surgeries and small surgical interventions, such as suturing, for example. Paresthetic symptoms in occipital neuralgia appear in the area of the occiput and may appear separately from pain.

Hyperalgesia – The opposite of allodynia, this is a symptom of pain that is provoked with stimuli that are normally inducing pain, but the pain is amplified (*hyper*). However, they are often combined. There is increased sensitivity to stimuli in order to protect the tissue from further damage and promote healing. Hyperalgesia and allodynia are both induced by substances such dykinin, prostaglandins, and substance P from the harmed and nerve. Hyperalgesia is a response to either damage to the tissue or damage to the nerve itself. *Hyperpathia* is a pain that lasts long after painful stimuli or painless activity.

Sudden (paroxysmal) pain develops in most people with occipital neuralgia. Pain lasts a couple of seconds or sometimes minutes. It is described by patients as an electrical-shock like or lightning-like. Pain is either sharp or dull, and it follows the pathway of the nerve. Sharp pain is in form of stabbing and burning. Sometimes pain is throbbing and dull. Usually the greater occipital nerve is affected, so the pain travels from the neck and occiput upward and toward the front of the skull. If the lesser occipital nerve is affected, pain spreads above the ear, and if the third, then the pain is located in the middle of the neck and occiput. Pain may become so severe that it affects other organs and systems as well, and it can be responsible for a sudden rise in blood pressure. This type of pain comes in repeating episodes, with the victim's fear and discomfort increasing with expectation of the next episode of pain.

Continuous headache is present all day, almost every day, and a person reports about having this type of headache for months or years. This is referred to as a *chronic* continuous headache. This pain is usually associated with muscle spasms. Pain is induced by chronic, prolonged improper posture of the head and neck, during sleep or the working day. The degeneration of neck structures develops over many years and, while this process gradually progresses, a person experiences pain that becomes more severe. Improper positions that a person takes are abnormal rotation or hyperextension. The pain may be on both sides but more often is one-sided. With chronic symptoms and muscle tension in the neck structure, pain may become accompanied with nausea, vomiting, or dizziness as the symptoms of an aura, much as with a migraine.

Continuous pain may develop suddenly, in a matter of days or weeks, and is called acute pain. *Acute* continuous occipital headache is often triggered with cold and lasts for about 2 weeks and then comes the remission (status improvement). It develops because of the sudden damage to the nerve. Both acute and chronic pain limit a person's ability and activity, and affect on professional and personal life.

Location of the pain – Pain is usually positioned on the back of the head, and is one-sided; however it is possible for the pain to appear on both sides. It is located differently depending on which occipital nerve is affected. Going from the midline to the earlobe and up toward the top of the head, a person may experience pain with some paresthetic symptoms. The pain spreads through the nervous pathway. Pain may move from one place to another, as a person moves the head and neck. It may spread to the temporal region and forehead and to the eyes. Sometimes, a person is convinced that he/she has problems with eyes, when actually they have occipital neuralgia. *Pain behind the eye* appears because of the specific pathway of occipital nerves. Sometimes the pain may spread to the teeth (dental pain).

Aura symptoms (migrainous-like symptoms) and *Sensitivity to light (photophobia)* may appear, as with migrainous pain. Other symptoms that may look like a migraine are *nausea, vomiting, dizziness, blurred vision, and stuffed nose*. These symptoms are called vegetative or autonomic symptoms and they appear as a reaction to stimuli that provoke pain in the head and affect autonomic nervous system in the brain at the back of the head. These symptoms may make occipital neuralgia look like a migrainous bout, when they actually have a different pathophysiology and treatment.

***

The intensity of pain needs to be adequately and objectively measured. Doctors use various scales to check for the intensity of pain symptoms, and effectiveness after treatment. A doctor may use verbal or non-verbal scales. Sometimes pain is divided into five simple categories: mild, moderate, severe, very severe and incapacitating, or simpler: no pain, mild, moderate, severe.

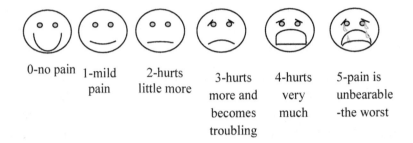

0-no pain   1-mild   2-hurts   3-hurts   4-hurts   5-pain is
            pain   little more   more and   very   unbearable
                                       becomes   much   -the worst
                                       troubling

Other doctors use more detailed scales for pain assessment. These include 10 possible answers, listed gradually from no pain to the pain which a person can't handle anymore, and maybe even passes out. Here are the 10 stages:

0 - no pain, comfort, good mood
1 – slight discomfort and disturbance
2 – pain is very mild, only noticeable
3 - sharp, short-lasting pain
4 – more distress and pain, manageable with medication
5 – pain that is sometimes severe, but with episodes of mild or no pain
6 – severe headaches with disturbance in normal functioning; tension headache is an example of sharp pain that a person handles with difficulty.
7 – migraine and cluster headaches usually have this severity of pain that comes in bouts, with gradual increase and decrease
8 – extreme pain, for example childbirth, that develops with huge changes in body and mind
9 – long-lasting, extreme pain, resistant to moderate pain-killers, and a person functions with difficulty; is usually followed by other problems as well, such as depression, loss of energy and appetite, and sleep problems
10 – pain is so severe that a person loses consciousness because of the huge amount of energy lost in the battle with pain and its cause

Chapter 6. Diagnosing occipital neuralgia

Diagnosis constructs the skeleton of any illness and facilitates the choice for the right therapy. This condition may appear like many others that are even more often common in population. Some are serious and some are not. Your health care provider will first make sure to exclude other diseases that have a worse prognosis and are potentially more dangerous than occipital neuralgia. That is why he/she will perform various assessments and may draw some blood from you to order some laboratory tests, before he sets any treatment for you.

Patient history

Your doctor will need to have a detailed conversation with you about when the headaches first started, whether anything you do provokes them (physical activity, food, medications), are you under great stress at work or at home, do you have any other illnesses, such as high or low blood pressure, heart condition, respiratory obstruction/infection, diabetes, problems with muscles and vertebral column). It is important what type of job do you have and for how many years you have been doing it. Some specific positions may have an impact on neck muscles, but stress is a factor, as well. We tend to take a specific position to defend ourselves from the threats and frustrations. He/she will ask you about how frequently do these headaches happen, do they appear gradually or suddenly, and how long do they last. How well you function in your professional and personal life may have an impact on quality of life. He/she will also be interested to know if the headaches have appeared before, what you have done to treat them, and whether it helped. People tend to use over-the-counter pain medications that are available to everyone. However, if the pain is neurological, these pain medications won't help. Family history may be of help to determine whether there is a genetic or some other predisposition for headache or increased pain perception.

The doctor will ask you about any problems with hearing, vision, instability in walking, and neck problems that could have been present from before. He will probably send you to some specialists, such as an ophthalmologist, physical therapist, ORL specialist (ear, throat and nose), or maybe a psychologist for help in dealing with stress and frustration.

Headaches may be divided into categories depending on their duration, onset, and provocation. If they last less than 15 days, we call them headaches with low frequency, and high frequency if it is more than 15 days. The individual episodes may last more or less than 4 hours. Based on that, they are divided into short- or long-duration headaches. People with occipital neuralgia often have problems with pain for several years before they visit doctor's office. The painful episodes are short-lasting but occur very often, with high frequency. (25)

	Low frequency	High frequency
Short duration	episode of cluster headache; headache triggered by high pressure in the head (coughing, exercise)	chronic cluster headache; chronic hemicrania in episode; headache during sleep (hypnic headache); SUNCT syndrome; occipital neuralgia
Long duration	migraine; episode of tension	chronic migraine; chronic

	headache	tension type headache; hemicrania continua (combination of migraine and cluster headache)

Clinical exam and nerve assessment

The doctor needs to know exactly where your pain is located, how it spreads, whether you have any pain triggers, and some other symptoms as well. He/she will most likely ask you what you do every day and what kind of posture you have during your working day. These factors may also influence the severity of your headache and associated symptoms. Then he/she will make an initial assessment, through clinical exam. Your neck might appear stiff and muscles are firm and tight, usually painful to touch. Pain may appear when moving the head in various directions.

The neck is a part of the body with many structures. If any of them is individually damaged, injured, or inflamed, it may cause some symptoms. However, not all of them induce pain in the back of the head. When he/she examines the head, he/she will probably find stiffness of the muscles of the scalp and maybe trigger the pain by touch solely. Besides the pain, he/she may provoke tingling, numbness, and shock-like sensation with palpation and tapping on the areas of the occipital nerves, which would prove the diagnosis. However, neurological symptoms are not necessary for the diagnosis but are facilitating factors in the diagnostics. If neurologic signs are present, a doctor may order some imaging techniques as MRI or CT.

The neurological exam includes palpation and percussion. By palpating the nerves on their pathway, the doctor may induce some paresthetic symptoms as tenderness and tingling. Percussion (tapping) of the pathway of the nerve may induce tingling along the nervous pathway, which is called Tinel's sign. This sign is positive in people with occipital neuralgia. (25) Another assessment your doctor may perform is with the pillow. He/she will ask you to lie down on your back and extend your neck and head backwards or rotate your head up until maximum. If the symptoms of occipital neuralgia appear, it is referred to as positive pillow sign. A health care provider may perform Spurling's maneuver, applying pressure on the neck by doing side and front flexion and hyperextension. By doing so, tendons, muscles, and nerves are being stretched, which may provoke pain and other symptoms of nerve damage to prove the diagnosis. This maneuver is also useful in other lesions of the cervical roots. (26) Electromyoneurography is rarely done to diagnose the location of damage.

Radiology (MRI, CT, vascular imaging)

If, during neurological examination your health care provider notices signs of nerve damage (paresthesia, severe pain, or some of the symptoms from the central nervous system), he/she is obligated to do some further analyses and advanced diagnostic radiological procedures to check for serious causes of such neurological signs. Usually, a person would be sent for an MRI.

An MRI (magnetic resonance imaging) is a radiological imaging technique in which a scanner uses a magnetic field to create images of the skull structures, but it can be used for all parts of the body. It can easily capture the soft tissue structures and abnormalities in the brain and other areas that may be responsible for the neurological damage. The causes may be tumors in the head, inflammation, bleeding, etc. If none of that is apparent, the neurological symptoms are due to other benign reasons.

A CT (computerized tomography) scan of the cervical spine develops images with X-rays and it can show the bone structures of the skull and vertebral column and their abnormalities that could possibly compress the occipital nerves. CT fluoroscopy with nerve block injection in the area of C2 nerve is sometimes considered the gold standard for diagnosis of occipital neuralgia, which is caused by entrapment of the C2 nerve. This procedure is performed in people whose pain is refractory to ordinary treatment and the cause has been found in C2 and C3. It is done with a nerve block through anesthetics in the area between C2 and C3. Guided CT fluoroscopy allows direct vision of the structures of the skull and vertebrae. The image moves as the fluoroscope moves. The procedure will be performed according to what a practitioner sees on the CT and the needle with anesthetic for nerve block will enter on specific places for C2 or C3. Some people may experience fainting after CT fluoroscopy, and other adverse effects aren't noticed. (27)

Vascular imaging may be useful to check for the inner state of arteries in the front and back of the neck area. These arteries (carotid and vertebral) are essential for the blood supply to the brain and other important structures of the head including sensory systems (eyes, ears, balance, etc.). If these arteries have blood clots in their walls and develop the process of atherosclerosis with progressive narrowing of the diameter of the lumen where blood flows, it can lead to serious problems because of the reduced nutrition. This can imitate the symptoms of occipital neuralgia. However, this assessment would need some other symptoms and is not considered as a routine part of the diagnostics for occipital neuralgia.

Ultrasound

The ultrasound technique uses sound waves that cannot be heard by the human ear to create images. It is useful for assessment of the soft tissues and state of the nerves that might be compressed with surrounding structures. With ultrasound it is possible to discover whether nerves are or aren't entrapped with muscles and, if they are, what the likely cause is. Ultrasound can be also used for therapeutic guidance when inserting the needle for nerve block through the skin to the nerve, and is much safer than injection guided by X-ray. (28)

Diagnostic nerve blocks and cuts

It has already been mentioned that blocks with anesthetics are used in occipital neuralgia. Sometimes the only way to a correct diagnosis is a therapeutic test that is, at the same time, a diagnostic test. This is considered to be a gold standard in diagnosis and the only way to determine exactly whether occipital nerves are affected and which one of them, knowing the exact anatomy of each one of them (even though lesser occipital nerve is sometimes duplicated, and not every person has the same distribution of these nerves). If, when injecting anesthetic, a person is relieved from pain, it means that the nerve affected with the injection is indeed a source of pain. The anesthetic causes deadening of the nerve and blocks the pain sensations from the nerve to the brain where we consciously receive pain. This procedure eliminates the pain only temporarily, for 20-30 minutes, and its only purpose is to differentiate the nerve responsible for pain. Corticosteroids can be injected alone in one injection to decrease the immunological response to the anesthetic and stimulate improvement. They are usually injected together. Some other diagnostic-therapeutic approaches include cutting surgically, injection of Botox (botulinum toxin that blocks the neurotransmitters from nerve to nerve communication), or burning of the nerve with radio-wave probe. All of them may be the introduction to the long-term therapy and are just introduced into the treatment to predict the effects they may have on the person. (18)

There are some side effects of such injection: infection, irritation, bleeding, pain on site, reactions from the needle itself, such as fainting, high blood sugar (which may also appear from the injection of corticosteroids), or allergy. It is, however, considered a safe procedure that is very useful in clinical practice.

Chapter 7. Occipital neuralgia and the differential diagnosis

Your physician needs to distinguish occipital neuralgia symptoms from many other conditions. Infrequently the cause of this neuralgia is a direct trauma, but more often the reasons are subtle damage to the nerves that respond strongly to the nerve blocks. Sometimes it is difficult to find differences between the two or three conditions because their pathophysiology is mixed. Most commonly, occipital neuralgia is confused with migraine and tension headache and with previously mentioned conditions and illnesses that present with pain in the back of the head. Here is how to differentiate occipital neuralgia from:

Migraine is a type of headache with specific characteristics of pain; it is associated with vegetative symptoms (dizziness, light and sound sensitivity, nausea, and possibly vomiting). Stuffed nose may be present in occipital neuralgia as well as in migraine. More severe symptoms such as light nuisance and vomiting are characteristic for migraine. People with migraine rarely report numbness and sensitivity of the back of the head and scalp to touch. This is characteristic of neurological etiology. Sometimes, people with migraine may develop pain in the back of the head, which is actually occipital neuralgia associated with migraine, with nerves affected (the greater occipital nerve). Thus, the symptomatology and the treatment become mixed. The only difficult thing is to distinguish the migraine and occipital neuralgia as isolated conditions and mixed migraine with occipital neuralgia. Some studies suggest that migraine includes some psychological factors in its development. Therapy for migraine includes treatment with triptans, beta blockers, calcium channel antagonists, ergot derivatives, and nonsteroid anti-inflammatory drugs and antidepressants. Nerve blocks will not bring pain relief in people with migraine, since the mechanism of development is based on cellular level hyperexcitability and not only nerve damage. Most of these medications are not effective in occipital neuralgia.

Tension headache doesn't share as many similarities with occipital neuralgia as migraine and occipital neuralgia (ON) do. A tension headache is usually mild to moderate, with pain that spreads around the head as a band. Dizziness, nausea, light nuisance, numbness, and a shock-like pain are more frequent with occipital headache. Tension headache tends to affect both sides of the head, while occipital neuralgia may appear on one side or both sides. When the pain and tension on the back of the head are dominant in tension-type headache, it may appear as ON. If this is the case, nerve blocks won't help and the cause of pain is declared as stress and lack of ability to cope with it. Usually, tension headache is declared as a myofascial pain, pain that comes from tension of the muscles, or compromised blood circulation. Thus, the treatment includes muscle relaxants but also antidepressants and anti-anxiety medications. Some studies suggest that tension headache is a type of somatoform disorder (physical symptoms appear for psychological reasons, as a way of channeling of the improper emotional expression, frustrations, and stress). This means that, psychological methods, such as cognitive behavioral therapy and relaxation methods, may play a role in treatment.

Cluster headache is a very painful type of headache that begins around the eye and is followed by symptoms such as red eye, swollen eyelid, sweating of the area above the eye and on the forehead, small size of pupils, drooping eyelid, and runny nose. These symptoms appear because of damage to and stimulation of the trigeminal nerve, particularly the supraorbital nerve, but there are other theories as well. A person who has cluster headache is very nervous and anxious about the next attack. Pain may appear as similar to occipital neuralgia since the pain from ON spreads to the back of the eye, but never with such intensity of symptoms in the eye as in cluster. In occipital headache, pain is also sudden and shock-like, but lasts shorter than with cluster headache. Cluster headache is sometimes difficult to distinguish from

65

migraine with eye symptoms of aura. However, migrai
associated with symptoms of the eye such as redness,
eyelid and similar, as a cluster headache is. Also, light and
sensitivity is on the same side as the eye with symptoms a
pain, which can't be said for a migrainous episode. In addition, a
cluster headache at the longest lasts four hours, while migraine
may last even days. A health care provider will probably order an
MRI to check the state of inner facial structures, the sinuses, for
example. There is a condition that is referred to as *hemicrania
continua*, which contains mixed characteristics of a cluster
headache and a migraine. Nerve blocks in the occipital region
won't bring any pain relief, which rejects the ON diagnosis.
Cluster headache is treated with mask of 100% oxygen,
sumatriptan nasal spray, Migranal, calcium channel blockers,
corticosteroids, and topiramate. (4)

Trigeminal neuralgia (tic douloureux) is damage to the three-
branch nerve of the head. It is the most frequently diagnosed
neuralgia of the head and face. The pain is usually located in the
area that is innervated by the lower branch of the trigeminal
nerve, the mandibular nerve. The key is that it characteristically
appears on the face. A person experiences one-sided pain in the
jaw and cheeks with neuropathic symptoms. Pain is sudden and
like an electric shock. It is easily differentiated from occipital
neuralgia. But, if the pain from affected greater or lesser occipital
nerve spreads to the side of the head, there is a problem in
diagnosis and differentiation between the two. However, pain in
trigeminal neuralgia never spreads to the rear of the head. Nerve
block is useful to find the nerve that is affected.

Myofascial pain syndrome is a pain that originates from the
muscles. Often there are trigger points, which, when pressed,
provoke moderate to severe pain on the site but on distant places
as well. Pain is spread through the *fascia*, which is the outer,
protective layer of the muscle. Usually the muscles that receive
the most pressure are the muscles of the neck and back. Muscles
of the neck may become stiff and painful to touch, and pain may
spread to the back of the head and all the way to the scalp, similar

to occipital neuralgia. Pain spreads almost immediately and is tension-like. Muscles are sensitive to touch and pressure. Therapy is conservative, with attempts at pain medication and antidepressants, and also some physical therapy methods, such as massage, exercise, improving the posture of the body, acupuncture, and heat, locally applied in order to promote circulation and improve healing. Usually the combination of these conservative methods brings definite relaxation and release pressure from the muscles.

Cervical facet syndrome (CFS) has symptoms that are very similar to occipital neuralgia. The main cause of pain is the degenerative process in the joints between the posterior parts of vertebrae that are important for the extension of the neck. This condition may actually be the cause of occipital neuralgia but, according to some guidelines, it may be a separate condition with its wn therapeutical approaches. Occipital neuralgia always includes neurological damage and neurological symptoms, which doesn't necessarily happen in cervical facet syndrome. Symptoms of CFS are tenderness and pain in the area of the joint, pain that appears with movement, especially extension and rotation of the neck, and is described as dull and with discomfort. People with occipital neuralgia may also have difficulties with moving the head and neck. It is difficult to differentiate the two, but degeneration of structures in CFS may be seen on the X-rays and on CT. The two conditions have different therapy approaches: CFS is treated with physical therapy (kinetic therapy and others), and occipital neuralgia is often treated with anesthetic injections. The two should also be distinguished from migraines and tension headache. (29) Nerve blocks may not be enough for diagnosis, since the occipital nerves may be affected if the C2 nerve root is affected. That is why your health care provider will most likely do the radiological procedures.

Herpes zoster (shingles) is a condition that presents with sharp pain and tenderness, numbness, and tingling along the nerve pathway; blisters and crusts form on the area of skin above the nervous pathway. Shingles is caused by the varicella zoster virus.

67

After chickenpox infection in childhood, the virus stays in the organism, in the nervous ganglions, until the immunity drops due to older age or an illness. Only then, the Varicella-zoster virus comes out from the ganglia and through the nervous pathway of some nerve, comes to the skin and induces the skin symptoms, along with neuralgia. The neuralgia may appear in the area of the nerves of the face and it may be severe and may last for weeks and months to come. However, the specific results of neurological assessment show whether it is occipital neuralgia or herpes zoster, even though in many cases the diagnosis is clear with appearance of the rash and blisters and crusts. It is, however, rare. Herpes zoster usually appears in other places (in ear canal, on the upper part of the face, or on the torso). Herpes zoster is best treated with symptomatic therapy, pain-killers, anti-itching medication, baths, powders, and boric acid.

Cervical myelitis or cervical spondylotic myelopathy is a condition in which there is damage to the spinal cord; the reason for this usually lies with arthritis or spondylosis (damage to the spine that occurs with aging, disc degeneration, degeneration of the joints, or degeneration of the bones). The symptoms are not limited to the neck and back of the head, but appear on arms and legs as well, possibly along with tenderness, numbness, weakness of arms, leg stiffness, loss of balance, and problems with urination. These symptoms appear as more severe than in occipital neuralgia and are often treated with surgery or powerful interventions. Occipital neuralgia is only limited to the head, which differentiates it from CM.

Inflammation of the occipital artery is a theoretical possibility for the cause of compression on the occipital nerve. The inflammation is called vasculitis, and it appears for known and unknown reasons. The symptoms include pulsating pain, maybe some swelling, mild pain. There won't be a response on nerve blocks, unless the inflamed artery begins to pressure the greater occipital nerve and cause its damage.

Eagle's syndrome is present in people who have an abnormally long styloid process, a part of temporal bone of the skull, which is located on both sides of the throat. This process compresses surrounding structures, where there is a complex web of nerves and arteries. Any nerve may be affected, the 10th, 11th or 12th or some of the branches. The nerve is mechanically affected by the bone process and it can be the cause of pain in the throat and mouth. Besides pain deep in the head, a person may experience buzzing in ears, pain behind ears, sensation of something being in the throat, change in voice, or pain in the face while moving the head. This may look similar to the pain in the back of the head. The treatment may be surgical to remove the part of the bone or to release the ligament which could also have the same clinical picture.

Tumors of the head or neck may compress the occipital nerves, and this includes much more severe neurological symptoms than the neuralgia itself. The health care provider would have to eliminate or prove this as a diagnosis with MRI. Tumors develop over the years, so the symptoms must develop slowly. Tumors that may appear in this region are either benign or malignant. Often the tumors are meningiomas that grow on the rear part of the brain (from outer layers of the brain-meninges), and other tumors may be metastases from anywhere in the body.

Other differential diagnoses include whiplash injuries and innate malformations (Chiary). Whiplash may actually play a role in the development of occipital neuralgia, but are not considered to cause it directly. Pain may also appear from the surface of the skin, which is physically injured or suffers some form of infection. Both of the two would appear with specific signs on the skin. Pain from the increased or low blood pressure is according to studies connected to otherwise present predisposition for headaches. If nerve blocks are performed in any of these conditions, they are less likely to be effective.

Chapter 8. Occipital neuralgia treatment

Occipital neuralgia is a treatable and in many cases successfully manageable condition. Prognosis is good. There are, however, people whose occipital neuralgia is refractory to ordinary treatment options. But there are still other approaches even for them. Treatment is either surgical or conventional and symptomatic. Some patients require interventions and procedures that are repeatedly performed in order to maintain painlessness. Depending on how far the diagnostic procedures have been conducted, and what the findings were, people receive different treatment. If the cause of occipital neuralgia is structural, which means that a structure such as a tumor, for example, compresses the nerve, there is a need for surgical extraction in order to relieve symptoms. Many people with this condition actually don't have any structural cause, but rather some cause that often remains undiscovered. These neuralgias are treated conservatively, with medication or nerve blocks, which is considered the gold standard.

Medical (pharmacological) treatment

The first line of treatment, at home, is the relief of pain with ordinary medications intended for mild to moderate type of pain. These are over-the-counter medications that are easy to acquire. Pharmacological treatment is not effective in many people. It includes only using pain medications to relieve pain but, if there is a pressure on the nerve, the symptoms remain until the obstruction is handled. However, there are many types of medications for pain. Typical types of tablets that are commonly used when there is a pain are aspirin or acetaminophen. These medications are of little or no use to people with neuralgia. Nerves react to various kind of medication. Antidepressants and antiepileptics (anticonvulsives) are the medications that have good effect in treating pain in neuropathy, even though their names suggest treatment of other diseases as well. It was discovered that they can also modify neurological response in the formation of pain signals to the brain. In addition, there are substances, not ordinary medications, that are confirmed as beneficial in treatment of occipital neuralgia.

1. *Zostrix* (capsaicin 0,025%), over-the-counter (available without prescription) pain relief cream. Its mechanism is to eliminate the substance P from the pain site, which is one of the substances responsible for the creation of pain stimuli. Capsaicin also lowers the production of substance P after prolonged use. It is also a muscle relaxant so, in any condition where muscles are under tension and stiff, it may be useful to try it out. It is applied 3-4 times a day. It has been proven that capsaicin is effective even after only one application for 60 minutes, relieving pain for the next 12 weeks. Capsaicin is produced in form of transdermal patches, creams, and gels. It doesn't absorb well through the skin, which is good and minimizes the chance of any systemic adverse effect. The use of Zostrix cream involves application of a thin layer, followed by massage. It is important to wash hands after use, and not to touch sensitive parts of body, especially the eyes. The cream induces a warm sensation on the skin, but that is the effect that works. Improvement of circulation with heat is beneficial for healing and muscle relaxation. It is often advised to use it after some other medications aren't helping. Do not use it if you are allergic to capsaicin. Side effects that can be expected include warmth and burning on site and a doctor's advice is needed when these symptoms last long or worsen. Other adverse effects are coughing, sneezing, irritation, allergic reactions. (30)

2. *Anesthetics* – Xylocaine and 5% lidocaine are anesthetics that can sometimes be used for treatment of occipital neuralgia. Anesthetics provide pain relief with various mechanisms that work on the cellular level and regulate electrical transmission between the nerves. They induce numbness and "deactivate" nerve signals to the brain. Their effect depends on the type and dosage of anesthetic.

EMLA 5%, which contains 2.5% lidocaine and 2.5% prilocaine, is a cream that can be also used locally. Ketamine is used in form of a lotion. A lidocaine patch (5%) is used as a form of treatment at the surface of the skin. (31) Side effects of local anesthetics include abnormal skin reactions such as irritation, burning, and redness, allergic reactions, difficulty in breathing, lightheadedness, euphoria, dizziness, tinnitus, vomiting, and some others. These products may include other substances, for example, aloe vera. If allergic to anesthetics or any adjuvant substance, do not use.

3. *Aspirin* – Acetylsalicylic acid (ASA) is an analgesic that can be used to calm the pain. It is often the first line of medication used whenever there is pain in any part of the body. Its mechanism is to decrease the production of prostaglandins that mediate in the process of inflammation and pain. Aspirin is only used temporarily for treatment of mild to moderate pain. Because of its possible side effects, it shouldn't be used in a long-term therapy. Adverse effects include bleeding in the gastrointestinal system and possible bleeding on other sites as well, dizziness, tinnitus, and allergic reactions. It is not recommended in pregnancy or for children under the age of 12. Since these medications do not have positive effects on many people with occipital neuralgia (or neuralgia in general), it is better to use other medications, such as antidepressants and anticonvulsives. Their mechanism of action doesn't include any effect on neurologic transmission. That is why they are ineffective unless there is an inflammation to the tissue.

4. *Acetaminophen* (paracetamol) is a drug that is used for relief of pain and high fever. Acetaminophen helps in mild to moderate headaches and may sometimes help in occipital neuralgia as well. It is used in form of tablets. Side effects of acetaminophen are allergic reactions, some liver problems that can manifest with jaundice, itching, dark urine, clay colored stools, stomach pain, loss of appetite, nausea. However, these are very rare and are

linked to high dosages. It shouldn't be used in people who have liver illness. If allergic to acetaminophen, do not use it. However, like aspirin it is often the first line of defense against pain, and it has fewer adverse effects, but is less effective than the specific medications.

5. ***Nonsteroid anti-inflammatory drugs (NSAIDs) and non-opioid drugs*** are medications that calm the inflammation, wherever it is, and include all of the other anti-inflammatory drugs, besides corticosteroid hormones, that are sometimes used for inflammation. NSAIDs are widely used in form of tablets, creams, or gels, for local treatment of pain. Most commonly used are diclofenac, ibuprofen, ketoprofen, naproxen, ketorolac. The mechanism of action is similar to that of aspirin. Sometimes, aspirin is included in this group. NSAIDs are used for pain and high fever, and in any case where there is inflammation. They do not bring great success in treatment of occipital neuralgia, since the mechanism doesn't include any modification of neurological response. There are NSAIDs with fewer adverse effects that are called COX2 inhibitors, which are used solely for joint pain. Some adverse effects are similar to ASA, and these are: heart attack, stroke, bleeding, ulcers, headaches, dizziness, buzzing in ears, liver or kidney problems, allergic reactions, and high blood pressure. NSAIDs shouldn't be used if there is allergy to them. In fact if a person is allergic to one medication from this group, it is good to avoid using any of them.

6. ***Opioids*** are medications that are used for treatment of severe to very severe pain that is resistant to non-opioid drug treatment (i.e., all of the previously mentioned pain medications). These medications use powerful substances whose basis is morphine, with its adverse effects (sedation, respiratory problems, constipation, nausea, and vomiting). Among these medications are morphine itself, fentanyl, oxycodone, hydromorphine, and meperidine. Their mechanism of action includes a direct effect on the central nervous system, with an increase in normal body analgesics that decrease the pain sensation. However,

these medications induce tolerance and addiction and serious withdrawal syndrome (after sudden stop in usage) and are only used for some people. In occipital neuralgia, they are only indicated for severe pain caused by either tumors or serious traumas. They, too, don't act on mechanism of neurological response.

7. *Muscle relaxants* are medications that affect the junction between the nerves and muscle cells and lower the contractions and tone of the muscle. This way the muscle is released from tension and becomes less stiff, facilitating regeneration and healing and releasing the nerve from pressure. Other muscle relaxants act directly on the central nervous system to relieve from spasms. This may be useful in spasms of the neck muscles during prolonged sitting in uncomfortable position, which causes mild inflammation of the muscles and stiffness, both of which compress the occipital nerves. Commonly used muscle relaxants are baclofen, chloroxazone, carisoprodol, cyclobenzaprine, dantrolene, and others. However, baclofen proved to be the only one that actually helps in neuralgia. Potential side effects include dry mouth, addiction, dizziness, and urine retention. The use of botulinum toxin as a muscle relaxant will be discussed later. Muscle relaxants can be used alone or with Carbamazepine (anticonvulsive).

8. *Antiepileptics (anticonvulsants)* are also used for epilepsy and disorders with convulsions, for neuralgias and neuropathies. After some of the medications from this group showed undesirable side effects in the treatment of epilepsy, researches tried to find different uses for them. Anticonvulsants inhibit the transmission of neurotransmitters, which transport pain signals to the brain. They increase the amount of GABA neurotransmitter, which has a role in neurological transmission: It calms down transmission, including the transmission of pain sensations. They are responsible for modulation of nerve response and have proven to be beneficial in neuralgia treatment. They can influence

neuropathic pain and other types of pain, including the previously mentioned influence on nocioceptive pain from inflammation or damaged tissue. The most commonly used are Gabapentin, Pregabalin, Carbamazepine Lamotrigine, Phenytoin, and Topiramate. Gabapentin (300-3600mg/day) and Pregabalin showed to be the most effective in the treatment of neuropathy. No specific blood testing is required while using Gabapentin and adverse effects proved to be tolerable. Carbamazepine (400-1200mg/day) is also frequently used to reduce pain in neuropathies but has different mechanism of action. (32) Lamotrigine and Phenytoin showed very modest effects, and are therefore rarely used. Treatment usually begins with small dosages and is gradually increased. Usually treatment doesn't begin with anticonvulsives, but rather with antidepressants. The first line of treatment from the group of anticonvulsives is however, Gabapentin. Possible side effects of anticonvulsives are dizziness, drowsiness, tremor, dry mouth, blurred vision, erectile dysfunction, swelling, weight gain, and anxiety.

9. *Antidepressants*, especially tricyclic antidepressants (amitriptyline), showed good effects in treatment of people with occipital neuralgia. They are considered as the first line of treatment. Tricyclic antidepressants (TCAs) deserve their name for their structure with three cycles. They were previously widely used in treatment of depression, but antidepressants have developed more and more, throwing TCAs into the shadow, so they found a new purpose in treating neuralgia. Even though they are antidepressants, they are used for various other conditions, including neuralgia. Their mechanism of action is to increase the level of serotonin and norepinephrine, but their effect on pain relief in neuralgia is not clear. Serotonin is considered a facilitating substance in our bodies that is a natural analgesic. Sometimes for them to take effect, 2-3 weeks need to pass, which is why it is important to stay patient and wait for the results. If it proves to be ineffective after 2-3 weeks, some other may

be suggested. Possible side effects include dry mouth, dizziness, nausea, blurred vision, problems with urination, excessive sweating, weight gain or loss, tremor, erectile dysfunction, diarrhea, and abdominal pain. Dizziness and drowsiness are reasons why these medications are used before sleeping and never before driving. They can induce seizures in people with epilepsy. A possible side effect of combined use with other serotonin-increasers is serotonin syndrome. It is important to get advice from your doctor about possible medication interactions. Another two antidepressants used for neuropathy and neuralgia are duloxetine hydrochloride and Venlafaxine, members of the group of medication called serotonin-norepinephrine reuptake inhibitors (SNRI). Duloxetine has shown excellent effects. They have similar mechanism of action and adverse effects as TCAs, but their side effects are much more acceptable than with TCAs. There are medicines that are now the first choice for depression but showed good effects in neuralgia too, the SSRI (selective serotonin reuptake inhibitors). They too increase the level of serotonin. Even though they are often prescribed as a first line of medication, they have too many adverse effects, which should be also considered. These medications induce depression or some unpleasant adverse effects in some people, and that is why there are limitations to their use. Anytime these medications are uncomfortable for use, it is better to perform nerve blocks or other procedures that don't require taking tablets.

General nerve blocks

General nerve blocks include injections of the anesthetic agent around the greater or lesser occipital nerve, in order to induce numbness of the sensory nerves, block transmission of pain, and decrease inflammation. Injecting agents to induce nerve block improves condition and relieves pain with unknown specific mechanisms.

Injection is performed in a clinic that specializes in pain o headache or in a neurology center. It is performed for the treatment of headache due to occipital neuralgia and also for migraine and cervicogenic headache. The effects are only temporary and treatment needs to be repeated.

The procedure takes only a couple of minutes. Here is how it is performed: The patient is placed in a sitting position with arms comfortably in front of them on the table. A physician prepares the injection with the chosen anesthetic agent. He/she will inject it in the area of the occipital nerve, which will result in pain relief for the next 12 weeks or so. In order to find the correct nerve, the health care provider may use simple palpation of the painful area or ultrasound or X-rays as a guiding technique. Some practitioners use previously described CT fluoroscopy as a guiding technique. The safest is to use the ultrasound to guide the needle to the nerve. There are many anatomic variations of the occipital nerves among our population. First, depending on the location of the pain, he/she will suspect which one of the three occipital nerves is most likely to be the cause of occipital neuralgia. If the first place of the injection is around the greater occipital nerve, he/she will do the following: the injection will be performed at one-third of the distance (about 2 cm) between the occipital's most prominent part and the mastoid part of the temporal bone, behind the earlobe. In this area, the occipital artery lies, whose pulse can be easily felt, and the physician must be very careful not to harm it. The needle enters through the skin and some deep tissue, so it is a little bit painful but, around the site of injection, the practitioner may choose to apply a local anesthetic. First, he/she will clean the skin area where the needle will prick with cotton swab soaked in a disinfection agent (alcohol). Then injection is performed. Your health care provider may choose to inject in the area on the line that connects the middle part of the ear lobes. The purpose of the first injection is to locate the specific nerve responsible. If the procedure on the

77

greater occipital nerve doesn't bring pain relief, he/she will try with an injection around the lesser occipital nerve. The injection is performed a little toward the earlobe from the site of the greater occipital nerve. The agent that is injected contains anesthetic (lidocaine or bupivacaine) and usually also corticosteroids (triamcinolone, dexamethasone, or methylprednisolone 20-40 mg), but they have proved to have some adverse effects if absorbed into the blood stream. The injecting procedure takes a couple of minutes and isn't painful. Immediately after the injection or in the range of 20-30 minutes comes the pain relief. The effects are temporary, however, and wear off in couple of hours, thus requiring repetition. Corticosteroids are applied for their anti-inflammatory effects around the nerve because, after the injection, a foreign body or anesthetic agent may provoke inflammation on site and steroids prevent that. The first performed procedure may be diagnostic/therapeutic to find out whether the occipital nerves are the ones causing the headache. If the status doesn't improve after injection around all three nerves, another procedure won't be done, since it wouldn't be helpful. If the injection works and brings immediate relief, there are open possibilities about further injections, radiofrequency methods, and implantation of the neurostimulator, because this way it is proven that the cause lies in the occipital nerves. After the procedure, the patient needs to sit comfortably in a chair and relax for a while. It could be helpful to apply ice on site.

Every fifth person experiences complete relief from pain and 50% of them reported that the pain decreased in intensity. The procedure is considered painless by many patients. The duration of its effect depends on the individual. Some people will feel numbness in the area for the next 24 hours and dizziness for the next few days. Usually the effects are more powerful and long-lasting if the pain has been mild to moderate and short-lasting before the nerve block. The first pain relief is due to anesthetics and wears off after a couple of hours; the effects of the corticosteroids begin to take effect after 3-5 days. Corticosteroids will decrease inflammation around the nerve, and provide effects that could last up to two months. The average duration is under a month and after that a person will require a new injection of anesthetics. How often the patient requires injections depends on him and the effects of the injections. Some need to have it very often and some rarely. Sometimes, in 15-30% of patients, the effects may last up to several months. Reinjection needs to be performed in 2 to 4 weeks, in order to maintain analgesia. If the procedure needs to be performed more than three times during six months, it is probably the best to find another approach for treatment.

With every medical intervention come risks and possible side effects. Side effects include some bleeding and swelling at the site of injection, which are mild. Some report mild pain on site and tenderness of scalp, and some even reported baldness on site after several uses. A person may experience some changes in their behavior for the first 24 hours and they should not drive a car during that period. (33) If a person is on anticoagulant therapy (blood thinners), or has infection, he/she should note that to the professional staff who performs the injection. If allergic to any of the substances used during the procedure, other treatments must be chosen. In general, it is considered a safe procedure. If the good effects of nerve block don't relieve pain, the diagnosis probably isn't occipital neuralgia.

People who have had occipital neuralgia for years before the procedure showed poorer response to nerve block, and those who had just recently begun having this problem respond excellently to the treatment. It is interesting that people who already used some medication previously in treatment of abdominal pain or migraines, such as a NSAID, have poorer effects than those who didn't. This is probably due to tolerance and increased threshold and the treatment needs higher dosages to work.

This procedure can also be used in surgeries to the head while awake. The principle involves injecting the anesthetic, which is usually bupivacaine or ropivacaine, and numbing the area of innervation of a specific nerve. The surgeon locates the nerve by knowing exactly how the muscles around the nerve are placed in relation to each other, and he/she must know where the nerves pass through those muscles. Some patients experience moderate to severe pain after nerve block. (12)

Occipital Nerve Block

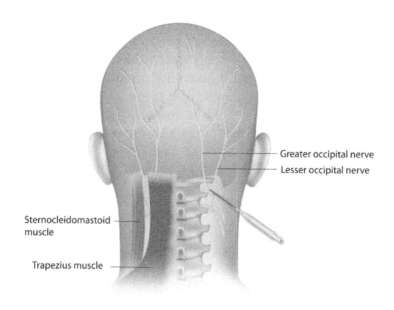

Greater occipital nerve
Lesser occipital nerve

Sternocleidomastoid muscle

Trapezius muscle

© Alila Medical Media - *www.AlilaMedicalMedia.com*

Figure 2 Location of the injection in the area of greater occipital nerve and position of lesser occipital nerve nearby.

Nerve blocks have also proven to be helpful in cluster headaches, migraines, and cervical headaches, with poorer results in tension-type headache and hemicrania continua. In all of these types of headaches, if a person uses analgesics that are becoming more and more ineffective, it is good to perform an occipital nerve block to provide pain relief in another way.

C2 and C3 ganglion block

There is a possibility of injecting anesthetic and corticosteroid hormones into the ganglion, which is connected to cervical plexus and occipital nerves, and to induce pain relief this way. The C2 and C3 block may also be diagnostic and therapeutic. C2 is located 2 cm from the mastoid part of the temporal bone, behind the ear, and C3 is 1.5cm below the C2. The procedure is considered comfortable and effective. The comparison of the two methods showed not much difference except for the frequency of appearance of pain, which was higher after occipital nerve block. However, studies show increased risk from systemic adverse effects, developing disbalance of hormones from the use of corticosteroids. But, C2 and C3 block also showed good effects and a pain relief that could last two months.

Surgical procedures

First, this does not include procedures that remove structural causes of neuralgia, but rather procedures that focus on treating the nerve and affecting the brain and pain sensation and perception. If there is a structural cause, the person is in need of open brain surgery and other specific treatments. If the reason is damaged nerve on surface, there are specific ways to approach it and accomplish good results in providing pain relief.

Surgical procedures are used as way of bringing pain relief to a more permanent phase. The patients who are not satisfied with the effects of current treatment, or whose pain is resistant to their effects, always have a surgical option available. Surgery is used to cut or affect the nerve, thus interfering with the transmission of the pain sensation. However, this may lead to the opposite: permanent pain. If the nerve is compressed, a surgeon will decide to separate the nerve from other surrounding structures.

Procedures that may be performed in order to bring relief are:

- Microvascular decompression

- Surgical liberation of the occipital nerve and neurolysis
- Rhizotomy and neurectomy
- Ganglioneurectomy

Decompression techniques and liberation of nerves

Whenever a tissue compresses one of the occipital nerves, or sometimes a blood vessel (this is called neurovascular conflict), the only solution may be to cut it and free the nerve. This is performed via microvascular decompression surgery. If an artery or vein compresses the nerve, surgeon will perform microvascular surgery. Compression by blood vessels has been proven as the possible cause of occipital neuralgia. However, when it comes to occipital neuralgia, microvascular decompression is rarely performed, because there are not many studies to confirm its benefits and occipital nerves are not frequently compressed with blood vessels. The position of those blood vessels and their spatial relevance to the occipital nerve is visible on MRI or CT. Microvascular decompression can only be done for occipital neuralgia if there is a firm proof seen on MRI. These are the patients that didn't have success in conservative treatment with medication and nerve blocks. They are the candidates for decompression surgery. (34) The procedure is done under a microscope or endoscope.

The whole procedure is minimally invasive. The incision is made on the rear of the head. Depending on what is compressing the nerve, different things will be done. The surgeon will follow the course of the greater occipital nerve and find the obstacles along the way. If the nerve is compressed by muscles, the surgeon will reposition them. If the blood vessel (occipital artery) that surrounds the nerve is compressing it, he/she will displace it. Lymph nodes can also be the cause of compression. This allows the nerve to recover and heal and regain its function.

The occipital nerve may become compressed by strong muscles, such as the trapezius, to such a degree that only surgery is a solution. Other muscles that may be the cause of the neuralgia are the semispinalis and the inferior oblique muscle. Neurolysis (liberation of the nerve) of the greater occipital nerve is performed along with cutting through the muscle. This procedure is performed in chosen patients who were confirmed with either nerve blocks or radiological procedures (CT, MRI). A surgeon will choose this procedure if there are clear signs of compression by the inferior obliquus muscle, or hypertrophy of veins around C2, or degenerative changes in the junctions between bones and ligaments that compress the nerve. Usually, they have problems with the greater occipital nerve and pain tends to increase with the head bending to the front. (35) (36) Rarely, the cause of occipital neuralgia may be the lesser occipital nerve and it too may be surgically isolated with neurolysis. The success rate in both operations is in more than 80% of the patients, with pain reduction in over 50%. This procedure has proven to be safe and with long-lasting effects. However, pain relief after this surgery isn't permanent, since the muscle may enlarge and regenerate and compress the nerve again. Indications for repeated surgery are less likely to be justified. (37).

Occipital nerves may become compressed by enlarged, damaged ligaments of the surrounding structures; for example, the ligaments of the joint between the first and second vertebrae in the neck (atlanto-axial joint). In this situation, the nerve may be liberated with decompression, bringing pain relief that can last up to 24 months, when there is a need for another surgical procedure. However, this type of surgery is helpful only in those people whose neck structures are responsible for the pain and sensitivity in the rear of the head. If the stiff muscles of the neck are responsible, a surgeon will perform liberation from the muscles. Patients will experience pain relief for a certain amount of time, after which the pain unfortunately comes back.

A patient is free to go home after one day in hospital, after careful observation of the effects. Some people take a couple of months to feel pain relief. The pain relief appears immediately and lasts up to one year after surgery in 70-90% of people. Of course, in some people, the effects may be only partial, which requires additional treatment with tablets. (38) (39) Side effects may appear and are a consequence of local anesthesia or allergic reactions. The most common are nausea and headache, which are temporary. Reasons for alarm are the following symptoms after the surgery: intensive headache, problems with sensation, persisting pain, swelling and bleeding on site. If the person isn't helped by decompression surgery, a surgeon might try with nerve section in chosen patients. This too may be followed with some adverse effects such, as numbness in the scalp area or lesser effects in those whose ON is due to neck disorders.

Another approach is with decompression of the C2 root and ganglion through decompression surgery. The incision is 2 cm long. The surgeon will free the ganglion and the nerve root from the compressive tissue or blood vessel. The posterior inferior cerebellar artery sometimes compresses C2 (there are cases in which the vertebral artery compresses the cervical roots and spinal cord). The procedure includes cutting in the area of the neck, just below the occipital bone. A surgeon needs to cut deep in order to approach the C1 and C2. After extracting a small part of skull he will see the course of the artery. The compression is due to its loop on top of the C1 or C2. A surgeon will then place polyvinyl chloride between artery and the nerve roots to isolate them from each other. Postoperative effects include pain at site, some bleeding, and numbness. This procedure may be combined with rhizotomy (discussed later), to increase the chance for good result.

This condition is often named C2 radiculopathy with symptoms of occipital neuralgia. Some doctors would think of it as a separate condition, which doesn't necessarily have to have an occipital neuralgia as a symptom, but it is mentioned here because of its close pathophysiology.

Rhizotomy and neurectomy surgery

Rhizotomy is a surgical procedure in which a nerve root is cut in order to relieve pain. This procedure was the first type of surgery proposed for the treatment of neuralgia. *Rhyzo* is a Greek word that describes anything that is connected to roots; in this case, nerve roots. The nerve roots are cut under general anesthesia, and the result is pain relief. Specifically, a dorsal rhizotomy on roots C1-3 is performed in refractory neuralgias. This surgery may lead to loss of sensation on the top of the head, numbness, which may be uncomfortable for the patient. (12)

Neurectomy is a partial nerve section. Neurectomy may be performed along with vascular decompression. The nerve is cut, thus blocking the sensory pain signals from traveling to the brain. This surgery showed a positive effect in 70% of patients that lasted for minimum 18 months. After that, the pain comes back, even though the nerve has been cut, in more than 50% of the patients and that is why this procedure is unsatisfying. There is possible risk for developing problems with sensation differently than before, increased pain and formation of a neuroma. In any procedure that includes cutting or somehow damaging the nerve to block its function, there is a risk for neuroma. Neuroma is a globule-like formation on a nerve, a result of tissue response and migration of the cells responsible for healing of the outer layers of the nerve. The neuroma can further compress the nerve and interfere with its function. It is the main problem that surgeons confront and it is the reason why some patients experience pain soon after the surgery and require second surgery. That is why surgeons developed other approaches and techniques to avoid the formation of neuromas.

Rhizotomy can be performed in the cervical roots as well, with a different efficacy rate. Another surgical approach is occipital nerve avulsion, which means "pulling." This means that the nerves are removed completely. Nerve avulsion has shown more efficacy than nerve section or some other methods. Then, medical researchers tried ganglioneurectomy.

Ganglioneurectomy

Ganglioneurectomy is a procedure much like rhizotomy. It is a procedure that involves surgery on the ganglion of the back roots (dorsal root ganglion, spinal ganglion) of C1, C2 or C3 that exit the spinal cord. This ganglion has an important role in sensation. It is a group of nerve bodies that form a globule-like structure. Ganglions are located on both sides of spinal cord, left and right. A surgeon may decide to do this operation after many others have failed to provide pain relief. Since the main cause of occipital neuralgia originates from C2, it is logical that the surgery will include extraction of the C2 ganglion.

It can be performed on one side or both sides, depending on the anatomical structure and cause. However, in this procedure the ganglions close to the spine are cut in the process of ganglionectomy. The surgery is performed with help of a microscope or endoscope. The ganglion and the nerve are cut. There are risks for possible inappropriate sensations, headaches, and postoperative complications.

Ganglioneurectomy may bring long-term relief to as many as 90% of patients, but the effects last only three months, with great risk after such surgical procedure. Removal of C2 and C3 dorsal root ganglions has proven to be efficient but is recurrent after a year in more than 65% of patients, which is successful but not an efficient enough result. (40) Removing the C2 ganglion was an idea that could actually work, since the lesser occipital nerve arises from it. It was developed after disappointing results from neurectomy, after which a neuroma developed and the lasting effect was short. Ganglioneurectomy showed good results but only in patients who have symptoms of sharp, shock-like pain, and stabbing, and it didn't show success if the pain was migraine-like (dull, aching, throbbing). This tells a lot about how the symptoms present depend on the cause of the occipital neuralgia, because both of the groups are considered a symptom of ON. (41)

These procedures that include cutting of the nerve or ganglion have sometimes no effect and, even though the nerve has been cut, the pain comes back. These procedures are considered ancient and, if possible, other procedures are performed instead. The new approaches that have brought an evolution in neuralgia treatment are radiofrequency ablation and nerve stimulation.

Radiofrequency ganglioneurectomy (RFGN), pulsed radiofrequency ablation (PRA) treatment

Radiofrequency procedures are minimally invasive procedures that include using radiofrequency waves to heat the tissue and thus induce dysfunction of the nerve. The procedure is performed under local anesthesia and with help of CT fluoroscopy. There are two types of radiofrequency procedures, continuous and pulsed.

Continuous radiofrequency ganglioneurectomy (ablation or destruction) includes destruction to the nerve responsible for headache, after it has been proven that it is indeed the correct nerve, with anesthetic nerve blocks. The radiofrequency method uses microwaves to "overheat" the nerve (denaturation). The treatment induces a low-intensity electrical field around the specific sensory nerve. Thus, the nerve loses the capability to send signals to the brain and inhibits long-term activation of the signals. The effects are beneficial and very effective as short- to intermediate-term persistence of analgesia. After the nerve has been destroyed, the pain may actually increase, which is the main risk of this treatment. Success rate is from 50 to 90%. (31)

The procedure begins with patient lying on his stomach, with the neck and back of the head exposed. The patient will receive muscle relaxants through a vein. The visualization of the procedure is obtained with CT fluoroscopy. First, the practitioner will wipe the place for injection with a cotton swab containing a disinfection agent. After application of local anesthetic around the area where the needles will be inserted, the procedure begins. Radiofrequency needles are placed on specific places on the back of the head and neck, depending on the position of one of the three occipital nerves. The depth of insertion is controlled through the profile projection from the fluoroscope. After that, through the holes where the needles are, a specialist will enter the electrodes and a low-intensity electrical current is passed through the area of the nerve. Corticosteroids are also used to prevent an inflammatory reaction to electrodes and microwaves. With electrodes, whose place has been previously checked on radiography, a low-voltage sensory stimulation is done. The targeted nerve is numbed with anesthetic (usually lidocaine) and radiofrequency creates lesions on it. The process takes 75 seconds. After that, the electrodes can be moved to other places to improve the effects. Some specialists withdraw the needles just a little bit and make another lesion that is more superficial than the first one. (42) This procedure is continuous and works through the mechanism of nerve destruction to provide pain relief. After the procedure, the patient may go home, but is advised to take a rest and not to drive. He/she may feel discomfort or pain on site. The effects will appear after 2-3 weeks, which is why it is important to be patient. There are some possible risks and complications to this procedure: permanent nerve pain, sensations of burning, pain at site, numbness, allergies, infections, and irritation of the nerve, which may induce symptoms such as sunburn. This procedure has shown some weaknesses in the shape of unwanted harm to the surrounding tissue. Also, with time a neuroma may develop, because this too is a procedure in which a nerve is damaged. After a while, the nerve will fully regenerate, and the pain may appear again. That is why there is a new approach, a new gold standard, pulsed radiofrequency.

Pulsed radiofrequency ablation is the newer version of the treatment for occipital neuralgia that includes radiofrequency. It is also used to facilitate nerve block effects. Other uses include muscle pain. The procedure is similar to continuous radiofrequency. Before the procedure begins, the practitioner will also apply local anesthetic. The needle is placed in the area around the nerve or the ganglion. It delivers short bursts of radiofrequency instead of continuous, as in previous method. It is applied in two pulses (or between 1 and 3) per second (20 ms) and changes the functions of the nerve, modifying its transmission of pain signals. Here the heat isn't used for the destruction of the nerve. That is why sometimes this procedure is called cold radiofrequency. The temperature at site is less than 45°. Instead, the nerve is restarted and reprogrammed into not sensing the pain. About 75% of people who had neuralgia in various parts of their bodies experienced improvement and better quality of life after pulsed radiofrequency ablation. Effects may last from six months to one year, after which the pain may become moderate again. Some people don't even experience benefits from this procedure. (43) Risks and complications are reduced by lowering the exposure to radiofrequency and heat. It is possible to feel mild pain on site or to have some bleeding. This procedure has been used for a couple of years and is not yet widespread, even though it has shown great results. People with occipital neuralgia are also yet to discover its benefits, because it hasn't been officially included in the therapy. Also, pulsed radiofrequency shows a financial benefit if we compare it to the continuous method.

It has been used in treatment of occipital neuralgia by taking effect on inner ganglion of C2 (dorsal ganglion), but there are potential risks of bleeding in the brain, and nerve damage, so peripheral radiofrequency is much more frequently recommended.

***

These procedures evolved from one to another, but neither of them satisfied the patients and relieved them entirely from pain. The only one that promises good results along with little or no side effects is pulsed radiofrequency ablation. Today, these surgical procedures need valid indications and are done after complete evaluation and assessment of the patient's condition. A patient needs to undergo some radiological imaging in order to understand the individual structures of the neck and a unique interposition between occipital nerves and surrounding tissue. A procedure that is at the moment considered to be the gold standard is the neurostimulator implantation, since it has shown very good effects and patients are satisfied with it.

Occipital nerve stimulator (ONS)

Nerve stimulation may help people with chronic pain. There are two types of nerve stimulation: spinal and periphery. This is the peripheral type. From 1993 to 1999, medical scientists were researching the idea of a stimulator that would be placed under the skin at the area of affected nerve to modulate the nerve function and pain perception in treatment of headaches. This would give neuropathic pain sufferers another option for treatment. In this procedure, an electric current is passed through the skin in order to induce pain relief. In 1999 they displayed the benefits of such a device in people with occipital neuralgia. At first, this device was tested in treatment of cluster headache and migraine. However, the device showed very good effects in people with occipital neuralgia.

The mechanism of action is neuromudulation, which is alteration of nerve activity through electrical or chemical stimulation. This means that the nerves that normally react to electrical impulses that come from other nerves are now being controlled from an outer stimulator. The stimulator interferes with the pain stimuli that reach the nerve and blocks them from further spreading to the brain, where perception of pain occurs. Also, the stimulator provides lower blood circulation, muscle and skin stimulation, effects peripheral neurochemical stimulation and the trigemino-cervical system, which connects nerves of the face and neck. The latter shows that placing the stimulator at the area of occipital nerve may be beneficial for treatment of migraines and other types of headaches.

The occipital nerve stimulator is a device with a lead electrode connected to generator that is placed under the skin to emit the electrical signals to the occipital nerve and then to the brain, with the purpose of hiding the pain impulses. It is considered the gold standard in therapy of occipital neuralgia. It is a type of neuromodulation in that the impulses are changed and modulated. A person is also given a way to control the flow of electrical impulses and thus to control the level of pain relief. Effectiveness of ONS can be up to 80% of the patients who were treated with this method. ONS is so effective that people report the headache was diminished and wasn't present in any of the following 90 days. To other patients who received ONS, quality of life was much improved and severity of pain was less after the treatment. However, ONS is not the first line of treatment and is also not effective for everyone, so it is only used for persistent, refractory, and resistant occipital headaches.

The procedure of implantation is done surgically in a hospital and the patient usually has to stay in the hospital for recovery and observation for the next 3 to 7 days. Usually, there will be a test implantation to check for the effectiveness in each individual case. First, the practitioner will prepare the patient for the procedure: expose the skin of the neck and back of the head, apply disinfection agent, and induce local anesthetic (lidocaine). Guidance is provided via fluoroscopy. The stimulator is placed underneath the skin, along the pathway of greater or lesser occipital nerve, usually on the level of C1. The place for the incision is either under the ear lobe or in the midline of the back side of the upper part of neck, just beneath the occipital bone. The localization depends on whether the nerve is the greater or lesser occipital nerve, which should be probably differentiated before this with nerve blocks. Surgeons have different results with the two approaches for incision, but they both showed good results. The implant functions with a special pad which a person needs to learn how to use. The pad is used for control over the level of pain relief. During those days after the surgery in hospital, medical professionals will adjust the level of pain stimuli according to each individual patient. The first stimulations are done as a way of testing the effectiveness. The procedure of implanting the part of the device that provides electrostimulation is done under local anesthesia. If everything fits and there is a good effect, a surgeon will insert the permanent stimulator under general anesthesia. The generator is placed either behind the collar bone (in the front chest; surgeons most commonly suggest this place), or on the abdomen, armpit, or buttock region, and sutured. The wires are connected to the area beneath the occipital bone. The batteries of the generator may be rechargeable and will last up to 10 years or non-rechargeable, which has a half of the other's lifespan. A patient is given a remote control device, with which he/she can reduce or enhance the nerve stimulation and intensity of pain relief and also switch it off or on. The new technology proposes miniature devices, bions, that promise better outcomes after the implantation, and easier manipulation, but the battery is much smaller and needs frequent recharges. (44)

Sometimes, when the person is home after the procedure, he/she may experience some trouble with functioning in professional life and while driving. The adjustment time may last up to 3-6 weeks. The device works on batteries that need to be changed every 1 to 2 years. Many patients reduce the usage of pain-killer tablets after the procedure in the post-operative period. This shows that the nerve stimulator indeed has excellent effects on neuralgia. If the stimulator doesn't improve the quality of life and relieve pain, it isn't allowed to remain permanently, because it won't be helpful. Many studies showed that patients who have undergone this procedure reduced the need for pain medication and felt better in general.

Side effects are relatively rare, but may appear as a consequence of an invasive approach. These are: lead migration, lead site pain, infection, contact dermatitis, pain on the battery site, incision site pain, neck stiffness, and possible risks that follow any other surgery and are a consequence of local anesthesia (33) A disadvantage of this procedure is that it is expensive.

Non-surgical treatments

Cryotherapy and cryoablation

Cryotherapy means "treating with cold" (low temperatures). With very low temperatures, a nerve becomes numb and the area becomes painless. This is widely known as a solution for pain. Applying ice cube on place where the nerve is causing pain or where it hurts will decrease the pain. The mechanism is as yet unknown, but it has been proven over many generations that the nerve is very sensitive to cold. The cold probably damages the outer layers of the nerve that are important for the nerve transmission of signals, and the sensations are not perceived in the brain. This we feel as numbness. If there are no transmissions of any sensation, then there are no pain signals to be received by the brain. Cryoablation means destroying with cold. The goal of this procedure is to destroy the nerve function with cold.

This procedure is done under muscle relaxation and local anesthesia. The guiding technique can be fluoroscopy or ultrasound. Before the intervention, the practitioner will have to determine through nerve blocks whether the occipital nerves are causing the pain in the back of the head, and which one is causing it. The rear of the patient's head is exposed. After cleansing the area with a disinfection agent and applying local anesthetic (lidocaine), the surgeon will begin by placing a small ice-probe (around 1.5 mm diameter) in the back of the head; this will create ice crystals at the end of the nerve and disable it. It freezes the nerve on temperature of 70 degrees below zero, thus blocking the nerve from sending signals. The substance that provides such temperature is nitrous oxide. Nitrous oxide is exposed to high pressure inside the ice probe, which creates the low temperature around the tissue. The entrance of the needle through the skin may be a little painful but it is short-lasting. The act is repeated in three cycles. The ablation takes 3 minutes with pauses that last 30 seconds and the whole procedure takes about 30 minutes. After this, the practitioner will also apply local anesthetic through the probe. The effects are long-lasting and cryoablation may be combined with nerve blocks. Since nerve blocks need to be performed very often, every couple of weeks, this is a good idea for minimally invasive treatment. Cryoablation offers a longer-lasting pain relief, even though the procedure needs to be repeated when the symptoms reappear. After the procedure, the patient is advised to relax at home and rest. Sometimes the recovery may take 1-2 weeks but, in general, the procedure is considered safe.

The effects of cryoablation last 7 months on average, but they may be maintained for 12 months. The nerve layers are destroyed to some point but they will regenerate after certain time. The cells of the outer layers have the power to regenerate, which can't be said for the nerve cells. This procedure may also bring some risks and adverse effects such as sensitivity to light touch, mild bleeding on site, infection on site, pain, damage to surrounding tissue, muscle spasms if in contact with the cold needle, damage to the skin from the ice probe, or, very, very rarely, neuritis, inflammation of the nerve, or even the destruction of the nerve, which can be avoided with specific measures during the intervention. (45) These adverse effects appear rarely, but are not uncomfortable. For only a few people, the symptoms of discomfort and numbness may persist for even two weeks.

Cryotherapy by cryoablation can be used in treatment of any neuropathy and neuralgia. Cryoablation has been shown to be more effective and with fewer complications than surgical neurectomy, where, after a procedure, the nervous tissue creates a scar-like structure, a neuroma that may compromise nerve function and prolong the pain. It may not be effective in people who have used antidepressants and pain medications for years, because some kind of tolerance has formed.

Botulinum toxin A injection (Botox A, BoNT-A)

Botulinum toxin is extracted from the bacterium *Clostridium botulinum*, which causes botulism. However, its effects are beneficial in medicine, depending on the type of the bacteria and toxin. Type A toxin was confirmed as a harmless and even useful substance provided by this bacteria, that might have a use in human medicine. Botox is used for various kinds of treatments, including esthetic surgery, treatment of bladder problems, and occipital neuralgia as well. It is especially reserved for people who had no luck with other therapeutic approaches in treatment of occipital neuralgia. Botulinum toxin is a muscle relaxant and nerve block agent and with those mechanisms is attempted in neuralgia treatment.

Botox A injection may be used as an agent to prevent the sending of pain signals to the brain. Botox does that by attaching itself to the cells on sites where neurotransmitters (acetylcholine) exit and travel to another nerve to pass the impulse on. If the botulinum toxin is bound on these sites, the neurotransmitter can't exit and can't pass the signal, so the muscle become more relaxed and there is no pain, consequently. Also, Botox A affects the release of the substance P, which mediates in transmission of pain, but also on calcitonin, a gene-related peptide and glutamate. Also, botulinum toxin has direct effects on the central nervous system in providing analgesia. This therapeutic approach is considered conservative and not invasive. Its effects are more lasting than the effects of other muscle relaxants. It can also be useful in treatment of tension headache and migraine.

The procedure begins after exposing the rear of the head and locating the nerves responsible for the pain. Botulinum toxin is diluted in 3cc of saline and injected into the regions of the pathways of either the greater or the lesser occipital nerve, into the area beneath the skin. Sharp pain in occipital neuralgia is eliminated for 6 weeks up to 4 months. Accordingly, people are improving their quality of life. (46) Possible risks and adverse effects include pain, bruise on site, inflammation, infection, or rash. Sometimes, if the needle hits a blood vessel and botulinum toxin enters the bloodstream, some systemic effects might appear that could trigger immunological response or hypersensitivity reaction. If there were similar reactions in the past, this procedure shouldn't be done. Also, pregnant women should take doctor's advice on using the botulinum toxin for neuralgia treatment, but it is probably the best to use some other procedure.

Phenol (alcohol) block

Alcohol injections have been widely used for treatment of trigeminal neuralgia since the early 20th century. Alcohol injections for this type of neuralgia helped in many cases and showed painless periods of, on average, 8 months. However, ethyl alcohol induces a burning pain at the site of the injection, and therefore, the use of phenol is recommended instead. Only a specialist in chronic pain may perform this procedure.

It can be used with some other substances, such as iopamidol, contrast agents, or local anesthetics. In the treatment of occipital neuralgia, researchers included phenol. This procedure is sometimes called chemical neurolysis because the liberation of the nerve and change of its structure is done with a chemical substance, with 4% or 8% phenol. Another type of chemical neurolysis is with iced saline solution, with or without anesthetics. Actually, these chemicals are used to prolong the effects of anesthetic nerve blocks, since their effect lasts for only a couple of weeks and, with chemical neurolysis, effects appear for much longer. For a proper place for the injection, the practitioner must locate the nerve that has been causing the pain. The procedure is guided with either fluoroscopy or ultrasound. Sometimes, local anesthetic (bupivacaine) is injected after the phenol. This is called a neurolytic block. A practitioner needs to be careful not to inject phenol or local anesthetic into the blood stream. The beneficial effects develop gradually, during the next 6 months. In that time, many patients reported that they felt great pain relief.

Phenol, although it has shown some good effects and is safe for many patients, has proven to do more harm than good if not performed by an experienced practitioner and has not been approved as a permanent solution for occipital neuralgia. There is a risk of severe neuropathic pain after the procedure and inflammation of the nerve. (47) Other possible side effects include dizziness, local tenderness, and drowsiness.

Physical therapy

This type of therapy may also play a role in managing neuropathic pain, since the muscles and joints that are included in the mechanism of occipital neuralgia respond to manual and other physiotherapeutic methods. There are various types of physical therapy (therapy with exercises, massage, electrostimulation, etc.) and they focus on relaxation of the stiff muscles and stimulation of the important spots that may decrease the pain's intensity. In order to successfully manage neuralgia, there is a need for a combination of beneficial treatments, which certainly can't harm if attempted.

Chiropractic adjustment

There are **manual methods** that are only performed when indicated. Some bodywork techniques may be helpful. For those people who have occipital neuralgia due to compression of some structure in the neck, there is benefit in manually repositioning the structures, and decompression. Of course, these are delicate procedures that should be always performed by an experienced specialist. So, basically, physical therapy can only help if the cause is in muscles or joints, the structures that can be modulated with hand pressure and mechanically reposition or circulation improvement. The muscles need to increase their mobility and they need to get their strength back to allow the proper neck movement without ailments. However, it is understandable that it isn't helpful enough if it is the only therapeutic measure, that is for sure. It is usually combined with pain medication or some other treatment options.

The chiropractic method includes, in addition to the previously mentioned actions, massage, heat and traction, along with learning the ways to accomplish healthy posture in everyday activities. Neck stretch is effective, and it may release the occipital nerve from pressure. Other exercises that your chiropractic practitioner might perform are neck rotation, neck extension, and flexion. Chiropractic methods include the person as a whole, trying to change the way our lifestyle and habits affect our health. Chiropractic methods work without masking the symptoms of pain. They might relieve from pain after whiplash injuries, consequences of improper posture, and nerve entrapment with stiff muscles. Along with those measures, a chiropractic practitioner might advise you to do other activities, such as relaxation and savasana yoga, and to have plenty of rest on a comfortable bed and pillow that is adjusted to your spine. (48)

Massage

Massage is used when the source of the occipital headache is muscle tension and stiffness after staying in an uncomfortable position for hours. This causes release of lactic acid and other substances inside the muscles, which induces pain, inflammation, and stiffness of the muscles. Touching the skin areas of these muscles induces pain in the neck and head. Massage of these regions may be helpful in people with occipital neuralgia. Muscles responsible for compression of the nerves and on which the massage can be performed by stimulating the trigger points are listed in following pages.

Trapezius muscle is the great muscle that lies on the surface of all the other muscles in the back of the neck. It controls neck movements and participates in arm and shoulder movement, as well. It is responsible for most cases of occipital neuralgia. It was previously mentioned that the greater occipital nerve passes through a channel in this muscle. Trigger points of trapezius muscle are 1) the place between the neck and shoulder joint; 2) the middle of the line that connects shoulder and neck; and 3) the place on the line between shoulder and neck and a little toward the spine.

Sternocleidomastoid muscle distends from the top of the breastbone and collarbone up toward the side of the skull. It is a strong muscle that can be responsible for various problems, such as dizziness and headache. Trigger point for this muscle lies along the whole muscle. Pain spreads from the back of the head and behind the ear to the front, to the forehead.

Semispinalis capitis is a small, strong muscle on the back of the head close to the spine. It is responsible for extension of the head and lateral flexion. The muscle may compress the nerves after a long time holding the head downward while sitting and writing or reading. Trigger points are located 1) at the junction of the occiput and neck and 2) at the middle of the neck, close to the spine, on both sides.

Splenius capitis muscle is a deep muscle in the back of the neck. It has similar actions as the semispinalis capitis muscle: extension and lateral flexion, and it is often strained after long time of reading and writing with the head bent down. The trigger point is located at the occiput just behind the ear and, when pressed, it provokes pain at the top of the head.

Suboccipitalis muscles are muscles that connect the bottom edge of the occiput and the vertebrae of the neck, C1 and C2. These muscles create the suboccipital triangle and are crucial in the development of occipital neuralgia. The occipital nerves pass beneath this triangle and, when they are inflamed, they can easily compress the nerves. They are responsible for facilitating the bending of the neck to the back and looking up. Trigger points are located at the top of the back of the neck in the middle area in the pit on both sides. When pressed, pain is provoked from the occiput all the way to the eyes.

Occipitalis muscle covers the occipital bone and is placed right beneath the skin. It can be responsible for the pain at the back of the head. The trigger point is located in the occiput and provokes pain at the back of the head and on the top of the head.

Digastric muscle is a small muscle at the front part of the neck. It distends from the chin all the way below the ear, to the mastoid part of the temporal bone. The part that is close to the back of the head is the trigger point of the pain that spreads from there to the back of the head.

Temporalis muscle is a flat muscle located on the surface of the bone at the side of the head. Depending on the part of the muscle that is sensitive, the pain may spread to the face, teeth, top of the head, or the back of the head.

Trigger points can be also the spots where a massage therapist performs the treatment to relax the muscles. A therapist will lengthen the muscles and apply pressure and then hold it. Massage of the trigger points needs to be performed at least 3 to 6 times a day, and can be helpful in relaxing the muscles, releasing the tension in the head and providing pain re. (49)

Warm compresses

Warm compresses may be used to improve circulation and facilitate healing of the damaged tissue of the neck. This method is simple and useful in everyday life. Usually injuries to the neck can benefit from warming up. There is still a dilemma as to whether it is better to use cold on nerves to numb the area or to apply warm and not hot compresses. Warmth can release muscle spasms and may make us feel more comfortable and relaxed. A warm compress can be made of anything; it may be simply a pad that has been soaked in warm water.

B vitamin nutrition supplement

Vitamin B12 is responsible for proper development and regeneration of the nerves, meaning actually the outer layers of the nerves. It is only logical that people with a neurological disorder such as occipital neuralgia may benefit from ingestion of B12. However, it is questionable whether it is good to increase the nutrition of such a vitamin after some neurolytic procedure. This is why it is probably the best to consult your health care provider about your state and how would you possibly benefit from the increased B12 intake. If damage to the nerve is severe, a person may receive B12 injections. This is characteristic of ischialgia. B12 may be ingested in form of tablets but there is also plenty of this vitamin in food. B12 is found in meat, eggs, milk and dairy products, fish, and fish oils.

Acupuncture or dry needling

Acupuncture is an ancient therapeutic method that originates from China. During acupuncture session, a specialist, the acupuncturist, will insert some fine needles into your skin. The needles are placed in specific places, depending on the organ or part of the body that is the source of symptoms. It was proven that, with acupuncture, nerves are stimulated, along with natural body responses and healing processes. This mechanism may be used in treatment of neurological pain. Some studies confirmed the benefits of acupuncture and acu-point injections. The effectiveness was 90%, which approves the use of this method as an adjuvant therapy of neuralgia. Dry needling is the Western-based needle therapy used on sensitive points of the body and is a modern, scientifically proven method, but it is very similar to acupuncture. With dry needling, a specialist will insert the needles in specific places of musculoskeletal tension or neuralgia, based on their position according to modern neuroanatomy. Dry needling stimulates the muscles and inactivates the pain. There are no chemicals injected, which is why it is referred to as "dry." Comparing the injection of local anesthetic, dry needling brings the same results but with more soreness after the procedure. Still, the researchers are yet to approve or reject such therapeutic methods and there should be more studies on this matter. (50)

Acupuncture includes actions that are performed on specific Ashi points on the body. These specific places are connected through nerve pathways and even the most distant two places in the body are somehow connected. Applying some massage or injection at the specific site induces good effects on the other part of the body. Specific places of Ashi points have to be known by the acupuncture specialist, who will know exactly how to perform this in order to induce positive effects on the body. Usually the tender points are the Ashi points for that region. After identifying the tender and Ashi points, the practitioner will massage the region and also apply some therapeutic needles which do not enter deep into the tissue. (51)

Cognitive behavioral therapy and psychological consultations involving pain and treatment

Since our minds are linked with nerves, such as the nerves that cause occipital neuralgia, it is only logical that anything that improves our mind-health can be beneficial for health in general. This type of additional therapy actually includes changes in the way we eat and drink, the vitamins we take in, how happy we are, and how often we exercise. But the core of it is in learning how to behave in difficult, challenging situations, and handling them without stress.

Chapter 9. Prevention

Since most people have had pain in the neck that transits to the back of the head and even to the scalp due to an uncomfortable position during work or sleeping, prevention focuses on proper position during these activities. If we think about the possible reasons of how degeneration of the cervical spine could happen, we still turn to the way we spend most of our day and how we sleep. We can protect our muscles, tendons, spine, and atlanto-axial joint by correcting the position of the head and neck when they don't move and when they are active. For example, when carrying some weight, not only are the arms under tension, but the neck is, as well. The position of the head depends on how heavy the weight is. When we are inactive, just sitting in front of PC, we don't move the head at all, which causes the muscles of the neck to hold the contraction for very long, requiring energy. That is when they become damaged.

These measures assure the correct position to release pressure from the neck, which is the crucial part of the body that presses the occipital nerves and C2 root. Of course it is probably best to dedicate some time of the day for exercise in nature and also to devote time for relaxation.

- When sitting, sit on a chair with arm and back supports. This way, arms are relaxed and the muscles of the neck, especially the trapezius, are not under such great pressure as when arms aren't supported and are in the air.
- The chair needs to be comfortable, but it is best if it doesn't have wheels, so that you can lean back freely, without moving away from the desk.
- When sitting, use a small box or a footstool to hold your feet on. This way not only the feet but the entire legs are relaxed and there is less pressure on the spine and the muscles of the back, as well.
- Your keyboard needs to be placed as low as possible so that your arms are not elevated and your neck is not under

pressure. It is altogether important that your computer is adapted to you and that you are not adapting your position to the height of the computer. Everything needs to be just within the reach of your arms and eyes, so that you are not bending your back. The center of the monitor should be at the level of your eyesight. If you can't change the table where your monitor is, there are monitors with adaptive heights. Also it is good if you don't have to move your head forward to read something on the computer or to sit in the crouching position where your back is bent forward and your neck holds the most pressure. The neck are of the spine is naturally curved but, with degeneration, it can with time become straight, which isn't good and induces pain in the neck and arms. This, too, is a reason to avoid crouching position during sitting. However, maintain the relaxed, tension-free posture.

- If you use glasses while sitting, adjust them to the distance from the monitor. The monitor should be 50-100cm from your eyes, so adjust the type of the glasses you will use if you use both reading glasses and glasses for short-sightedness.
- Sit with your back straight and move your head from time to time. You shouldn't hold your head in one position bent down and straight ahead. The same can be done while driving or sitting comfortably with friends. Always use good posture, which releases pressure from the neck muscles.
- Don't hold the telephone with your neck.
- Sleep in a comfortable position. Sleeping especially important since we spend a large part of the day doing it. Comfortable pillows and mattresses are important for the healthy position of the neck and back, which will provide resting of the muscles, without waking up in the morning with stiff neck. It is helpful sometimes if you sleep on your back, with proper neck and arm support, because this takes the tension from the neck, which reduces pain and lets the muscles rest and heal. Special neck pillows or

neck splints are used as a support for the neck. Actually, these neck supports can be home-made from towels or blankets.

- Do not fall asleep while reading or watching TV. This leads to pain after waking up. Some people, children mostly, watch TV while lying down, with the head raised above to watch the screen, but this leads to serious pressure on the muscles of the back of the neck and, most important, induces compression of the occipital nerves.

- If you already have occipital neuralgia, prevent further episodes of pain by wearing neck splints when falling asleep. You can also do this while sitting and relaxing on the chair. If you think you will fall asleep in the armchair while reading or watching TV, use a neck splint.

- Severe pain can be prevented by applying ice on the surface of the skin where the pain began and gradually increases in intensity. Nerves react to cold temperatures by blocking the transmission of impulses of pain to the brain.

- If the reason for the occipital neuralgia lies in the over-contraction of the muscles of the neck, it is more helpful to apply warm compresses, capsaicin creams, and anything that promotes circulation and facilitates healing.

- If you have sprained a muscle, prevent headache by treating the muscle before it compresses the nerve. Apply cold to calm the swelling or heat to improve circulation and healing. The muscles need to be relaxed until they are fully healed, and not pressured again. When sleeping, flex the legs to relieve pressure on the muscles of the spine and back. Muscles can benefit from massage. Apply analgesic gels (acetaminophen or non-steroidal analgesics).

- Exercises for the neck are certainly welcome, especially for those who sit for too long. Exercises that stretch and strengthen the neck are useful. Of more use are the exercises that include the whole body, by exercising the legs to reduce pressure on the lower back, and exercising the arms to reduce pressure on the neck.

In order to prevent the illness, we need to focus on the causes of the development that last either over a short period of time or over the years. Every measure that prevents injuries, especially neck injuries, will reduce the chance of having future problems with head and neck. If there has been a slight injury at work or while doing something, you may perform some measures to prevent the injury from going further, by taking pain relief medicines or creams, immobilizing it, etc. Other than musculoskeletal, reasons can be some systemic illnesses, tumors, blood vessels dysfunction, etc. If not improved before happening, these can be properly treated, with attention to good habits and lifestyle. Of course, some illnesses can't be controlled, but there are some measures you can take that don't induce harm and may even benefit you in stopping the progression of otherwise present condition. Staying properly hydrated, and eating well, with lots of vitamins, can be helpful. Hydration and healthy food are crucial in keeping the cartilage and discs between vertebrae elastic and durable. If you have a smoking habit, it is probably best to reduce it. Constriction of the blood vessels in the head may be a possible mechanism for headaches. If stress is the main factor in your life, use some techniques to relax. Even sitting in one position and not moving even a finger, with proper breathing through the nose and with your stomach, may reduce your anxiety and frustration level.

Works Cited

1. *Headache disorders.* s.l. : World health organisation, 2016. Epidemiology of headaches.

2. *Pain, Nicotine, and Smoking: Research Findings and Mechanistic Considerations. .* **Ditre JW, Brandon TH, Zale EL, Meagher MM.** 2011, Psychological bulletin 137(6), pp. 1065-1093.

3. *The brain is hyperexcitable in migraine.* **Aurora SK, Wilkinson F.** 2007, Cephalalgia 27(12), pp. 1442-53.

4. Types of headaches/migraine. *American migraine foundation.* [Online] 2010. [Cited: 1 11, 2017.] https://americanmigrainefoundation.org/living-with-migraines/types-of-headachemigraine/.

5. *SUNCT Syndrome: diagnosis and treatment.* **Pareja JA, Caminero AB, Sjaastad O.** 2002, CNS Drugs 16(6), pp. 373-83.

6. *Chronic headaches and the neurobiology of somatization.* **JM., Borkum.** 2010, Curr Pain Headache Rep., pp. 14(1):55-61.

7. **(IHS), Headache Classification Committee of the International Headache Society.** *The International Classification of Headache Disorders,3rd edition (beta version).* 2013. pp. 629-808.

8. Peripheral Neuropathy Fact Sheet. *National Institute of Neurological Disorders and Stroke.* [Online] December 2014. [Cited: 12 28, 2016.] https://www.ninds.nih.gov/Disorders/Patient-Caregiver-Education/Fact-Sheets/Peripheral-Neuropathy-Fact-Sheet.

9. Trigeminal Neuralgia. *NORD (National Organization for Rare Disorders), .* [Online] 2014. [Cited: 12 28, 2016.] https://rarediseases.org/rare-diseases/trigeminal-neuralgia/.

10. *Supraorbital neuralgia.* **Pareja JA, Caminero AB.** 2006, Curr Pain Headache Rep., pp. 10(4):302-5.

11. **Rubin M.** Glossopharyngeal Neuralgia. *msd manuals.* [Online] [Cited: 12 28, 2016.] http://www.msdmanuals.com/home/brain,-spinal-cord,-and-nerve-disorders/cranial-nerve-disorders/glossopharyngeal-neuralgia#.

12. *The innervation of the scalp: A comprehensive review including anatomy, pathology, and neurosurgical correlates.* **Kemp WJ, Tubbs RS, Cohen-Gadol AA.** Surg Neurol Int. : s.n., 2011, Vol. 2, p. 178.

13. *On the concept of third occipital headache.* **Bogduk N, Marsland A.** 1986, Journal of Neurology, Neurosurgery, and Psychiatry.49(7), pp. 775-80.

14. Suboccipital nerve. *Anatomy expert.* [Online] [Cited: 1 13, 2017.] http://www.anatomyexpert.com/app/structure/6551/22436/.

15. *Headache and hypertension: refuting the myth.* **D., Friedman.** 2002, J Neurol Neurosurg Psychiatry 72, p. 431 .

16. *Thyrotoxicosis presenting with headache.* **Stone J, Foulkes A, Adamson K, Stevenson L, Al-Shahi Salman R.** 2007, Cephalalgia 27(6), pp. 561-2.

17. *The Neuralgias: Diagnosis and Management.* **Gadient, PM, Smith, J.** 2014, Curr Neurol Neurosci Rep, p. 14:459.

18. Occipital neuralgia. *Johns Hopkins medicine.* [Online] [Cited: 1 6, 2017.] http://www.hopkinsmedicine.org/healthlibrary/conditions/adult/nervous_system_disorders/Occipital_Neuralgia_22,OccipitalNeuralgia/.

19. *Occipital nerve release in patients with whiplash trauma and occipital neuralgia.* **Magnússon T, Ragnarsson T, Björnsson A.** 1996, Headache., pp. 36(1):32-6.

20. *Neurological Manifestations of Systemic Lupus Erythematosus in Children and Adults.* **Muscal, E, and L. Brey R.** 2010, Neurologic clinics 28 (1), pp. 61–73.

21. *Vascular compression as a potential cause of occipital neuralgia: a case report.* **White JB, Atkinson PP, Cloft HJ, Atkinson JL.** 2008, Cephalalgia. , pp. 28(1):78-82. .

22. *Giant cell arteritis of the occipital arteries--a prospective color coded duplex sonography study in 78 patients.* **Pfadenhauer K1, Weber H.** 2003, J Neurol., pp. 250(7):844-9.

23. *Occipital Neuralgia as the Only Presenting Symptom of Foramen Magnum Meningioma.* **Kim, Nam-Hee et al.** 2009, Journal of Clinical Neurology , pp. 198–200.

24. *Allodynia and hyperalgesia in neuropathic pain: clinical manifestations and mechanisms.* **Jensen TS, Finnerup NB.** 2014, Lancet Neurol 13(9), pp. 924-35.

25. Occipital neuralgia. [book auth.] Hashmi M. Barna S. *Pain management rounds.* Massachusetts : s.n., 2004, Vol. 1 Issue 7.

26. **Singla AK, Silver JK.** Occipital Neuralgia. *Anesthesia Key.* [Online] 6 19, 2016. [Cited: 1 5, 2017.] http://aneskey.com/occipital-neuralgia/.

27. *Refractory Occipital Neuralgia: Preoperative Assessment with CT-Guided Nerve Block Prior to Dorsal Cervical Rhizotomy.* **al., Kapoora V et.** 2003, AJNR Am J Neuroradiol 24(10), pp. 2105-10.

28. *Occipital Neuralgia Diagnosis and Treatment: The Role of Ultrasound.* 2016, Headache 56(4), pp. 801-7.

29. *Cervical facet arthropathy and occipital neuralgia: headache culprits.* **JD, Hoppenfeld.** 2010, Curr Pain Headache Rep 14(6) , pp. 418-23.

30. *Topical capsaicin for pain management: therapeutic potential and mechanisms of action of the new high-concentration capsaicin 8% patch.* **Anand P, Bley K.** 2011, British Journal of Anaesthesia 107(4), pp. 490-502.

31. **Hain, T. .** Occipital neuralgia. *Dizziness-and-balance.com.* [Online] December 26, 2015. [Cited: 1 6, 2017.] http://www.dizziness-and-balance.com/disorders/central/migraine/occipital_neuralgia.html.

32. *Anticonvulsants for neuropathic pain syndromes: mechanisms of action and place in therapy.* **Tremont-Lukats IW1, Megeff C, Backonja MM.** 2000, Drugs 60(5), pp. 1029-52.

33. *Migraine and the greater occipital nerve.* Leicester : Migraine action, 2011.

34. *JB White, PP Atkinson, HJ Cloft, JLD Atkinson.* **Report, Vascular Compression as a Potential Cause of Occipital Neuralgia: A Case.** 2007, Cephalalgia 28:(1), pp. 78-82.

35. *Surgical treatment of greater occipital neuralgia by neurolysis of the greater occipital nerve and sectioning of the*

inferior oblique muscle. **Gille O, Lavignolle B, Vital JM.** 2004, Spine (Phila Pa 1976). 29(7), pp. 828-32.

36. *Neurolysis of the greater occipital nerve in cervicogenic headache. A follow up study.* **Bovim G, Fredriksen TA, Stolt-Nielsen A, Sjaastad O.** 1992, Headache 32(4), pp. 175-9.

37. *Indications and outcomes for surgical treatment of patients with chronic migraine headaches caused by occipital neuralgia.* **Ducic I, Hartmann EC, Larson EE.** 2009, Plast Reconstr Surg 123(5), pp. 1453-61.

38. Microvascular Decompression Surgery, Recovery Time, and Side Effects. *UPMC Life Changing Medicine.* [Online] [Cited: 1 9, 2017.] http://www.upmc.com/services/neurosurgery/brain/treatments/microvascular-decompression/pages/default.aspx.

39. **Neuralgia, Surgery For Occipital.** Surgery For Occipital Neuralgia. *drjasonhall.* [Online] [Cited: 1 23, 2017.] https://drjasonhall.com/surgery-for-occipital-neuralgia/.

40. *Pain relief after cervical ganglionectomy (C2 and C3) for the treatment of medically intractable occipital neuralgia.* **Acar F, Miller J, Golshani KJ, Israel ZH, McCartney S, Burchiel KJ.** 2008, Stereotact Funct Neurosurg 86(2), pp. 106-12.

41. *Microsurgical C-2 ganglionectomy for chronic intractable occipital pain.* **Lozano AM, Vanderlinden G, Bachoo R, Rothbart P.** 1998, J Neurosurg 89(3), pp. 359-65.

42. *Incidence of neuropathic pain after radiofrequency denervation of the third occipital nerve.* 2014, J Pain Res 7, pp. 195–198.

43. *Pulsed radiofrequency for the treatment of occipital neuralgia: a prospective study with 6 months of follow-up.* **Vanelderen P, Rouwette T, De Vooght P, Puylaert M, Heylen R, Vissers K, Van Zundert J.** 2010, Reg Anesth Pain Med 35(2), pp. 148-51.

44. *Occipital nerve stimulation in primary headache syndromes.* **Lambru G, Matharu MS.** Ther Adv Neurol Disord 5(1), pp. 57 - 67.

45. *Cryoablation for the treatment of occipital neuralgia.* **Kim CH, Hu W, Gao J, Dragan K, Whealton T, Julian C.** 2015, Pain Physician 18(3) , pp. E363-8.

46. *Botulinum toxin type-A (BOTOX) in the treatment of occipital neuralgia: a pilot study.* **Taylor M, Silva S, Cottrell C.** 2008, Headache 48(10), pp. 1476-81.

47. *Phenol Neurolysis for Severe Chronic Nonmalignant Pain: Is the Old also Obsolete?* **al., Weksler N et.** 2007, Pain Medicine 8(4), pp. 332-7.

48. **PK., Carr.** Headache-occipital neuralgia. *Dynamic Chiropractic Clinic.* [Online] [Cited: 1 19, 2017.] http://dynamicclinic.com/headache/.

49. **Psaromatis, M.** Trigger Points that Create an Occipital Headache. *Musle pain solutions.* [Online] 2009. [Cited: 1 6, 2017.] http://www.natural-solutions-for-muscle-pain.com/occipital-headache.html.

50. *Improvement in clinical outcomes after dry needling in a patient with occipital neuralgia.* **Bond BM, Kinslow C.** 2015, The Journal of the Canadian Chiropractic Association 59(2), pp. 101-10.

51. **T, Hendrickson.** *Massage for Orthopedic Conditions.*
Baltimore: Lippincott : William & Wilkins, 2003.

CPSIA information can be obtained
at www.ICGtesting.com
Printed in the USA
BVOW10s2003280917
496072BV00009B/343/P